AF655075

ENCYCLOPAEDIA OF AIDS

ENCYCLOPAEDIA OF AIDS

(In 7 Volumes)

(Volume 5)

Editor

Dr. G.C. Satpathy

PUBLICATIONS

KALPAZ PUBLICATIONS

DELHI - 110052

ENCYCLOPAEDIA OF AIDS
(*Health, Reference*)

Rs. 7000 (Set)
Rs. 1000 (each volume)

ISBN: 81-7835-112-9 (Set)
ISBN: 81-7835-136-6 (Vol. 5)

©Dr. G.C. Satpathy

All rights reserved. No part of this book may be reproduced in any manner without written permission.

Published in 2003 in India by
Kalpaz Publications
C-30, Satyawati Nagar
Delhi-110052
e-mail: kalpaz@hotmail.com

Laser Typeset at: Alphabet, Delhi
Printed at: Mehra Offset Press, Delhi

Contents

Preface

The later half of the twentieth century will be remembered in the history of medicine for two remarkable events, one good, that is the eradication of smallpox, and the other one bad, when the world was alerted to the first case AIDS in 1981, now running in a pandemic proportion. In a little over two decades it is estimated that over 36 million people are now infected with HIV/AIDS with 5.3 million being infected every year. India alone has about 4 million HIV/AIDS patients, the second highest number among all nations. Now it is well perceived as a serious threat to humanity, and the control of this epidemic lies not only in the hands of physicians alone but the entire society must involve to the task. No cure or vaccine is yet in sight. So the only mode of controlling it is prevention. The key to prevention lies in information, education and communication.

Twenty years of observation and study of the syndrome has generated profound interest among all branches of medicine, social activists, research workers, public health issues, health and sex education strategies, with innumerable clinical and pharmacological research being conducted on it all over the world. It is not possible to compile the whole saga of AIDS, which is unique in many ways and not yet fully understood. We have tried to accumulate as much information as possible in this seven-volume encyclopaedia, probably the first such attempt made ever. Since the process of acquiring information is never-ending, we hope to provide more and more information in future.

It has been a herculean task to compile the huge materials systematically, besides being an unique experience. In spite of the best efforts for accuracy and perfection, there may be shortcomings, which may be excused. It will be a success story for us if by this work the society to which the work is dedicated is benefited at large. The study does not end here. It shall be a continuous series in future with comprehensive details having a deep bearing on the subject.

Guwanati-23
Rathyatra-2002

Dr. G.C. Satpathy
MD, IPM

Acknowledgements

During the course of this research work, I happened to visit several academic fora which willingly afforded their support and facilitated my work. These are the Ministry of Health, Govt. of India, World Health Organisation, health departments of the States and academic institutions of higher learning. I have used the material from published works including scholarly journals and magazines to fill up the gaps in these volumes.

I have also taken academic support from several sources, which include universities, institutes, centres for higher learning, Acts passed in this direction, Statistical Year Book (UNESCO), voluntary organisations, legal luminaries, social activists, prison management, legal issues of AIDS, Legislation Enquiry Commission on HIV Law, Sri Lanka, Prevention of Brothels Act, Myanmar, Laws of HIV/AIDS in Pakistan, Documents in sub-Saharan, Africa, European Council Recommendations, UNESCO Courier, Philippines Overseas Employment Agency, Foreign Exchange Regulations Deptt., Central Bank of the Philippines, National Advisory Committee on AIDS in Singapore, Vietnamese National AIDS Committee, National Blood Transfusion Centre in Cambodia, Infectious Diseases Act, Thailand, AIDS Prevention Act in Korea, Labour Protection Law, Thailand, Social Security Act, Thailand, Homosexual Law Reform Act, 1986, Universities of Nairobi, Manitola (in Canada) and Washington, Institute of Systemic Therapy, Harare, Zimbabwe, The AIDS Service Organisation, Kampala, Uganda, Health Economics and HIV/AIDS Research Division, University of Natal, Durban, School of

Public Health, University of Natal, South Africa Institute for Medical Research, Johannesburg, Centre for African Family Studies, Nairobi, Kenya, Malwai Institute of Management, Malwai.

I feel much grateful to these institutions and learned authors whose writings have proved useful in the texts of these seven volumes.

The publisher and myself feel much beholden to the panel of highly qualified and experienced advisers who are distinguished in their respective fields, for their valuable and timely guidelines, contributions and encouragement in making this work an epoch-making one.

I am grateful to several other research institutes and NGOs etc., scholars whose writings have been used in these volumes.

I am extremely grateful to my wife, son Anurag and daughter Anamika for their consistent encouragement to me during this stupendous research work.

Dr. G.C. Satpathy

Our Distinguished Panel of Advisers

1.	Dr. A.K. Das, MD, MNAMS, Ph.D., FICA	Dean and Director-Prof. Dept. of Medicine, JIMPER, Pondicherry
2.	Mr. D.K. Arya IPS (Retd.)	Former Director General, BSF
3.	Dr. K.V. Dakhina Murty MD, DM, DNB, FISN	Prof. & Head, Deptt. of Nephrology, Nizam's Instt. of Medical Sciences, Panjagutta, Hyderabad
4.	Maj. Gen. K.K. Ganguly	VSM (Retd.)
5.	Col. M.K. Bhandari MD, FICA	Asso. Prof. of Medicine, Armed Forces Medical College, Pune
6.	Dr. M.C. Dash	Vice Chancellor, Sambalpur University, P.O.: Jyoti Vihar, Orissa
7.	Dr. N.C. Borah MD, DM	C.M.D. GNRC Hospitals Ltd. Dispur, Guwahati
8.	Dr. P.C. Bhattacharya MD	Sr. Consultant, downtown hospital Dispur, Guwahati
9.	Dr. S.B. Gupta MD	Physician and Cardiologist Central Railway Hospital, Mumbai

Introduction

The AIDS Network

As the epidemic of HIV/AIDS has grown, so have programmes and projects to combat it. It is striking that there are pockets of excellence in research and programme effectiveness, but that these pockets are outnumbered by less effective efforts that have much to learn from the successful responses. There is a need to make better use of the knowledge of what works against HIV/AIDS, to increase this knowledge base and to share it more effectively and efficiently. This book presents an illustrative framework for understanding how networks and networking add value to HIV/AIDS activities. It is a guide to effective networking for individuals and institutions working on programmes to reverse the course of the HIV/AIDS epidemic. It is mainly addressed to programme managers, network facilitators and others involved in expanding the response to HIV/AIDS, including UNAIDS co-sponsors, NGOs, bilateral organisations and multilateral agencies.

The Government and organisations or individuals involved in HIV/AIDS prevention, care, treatment and support activities need to have the skills, knowledge and experience to be optimally effective. In pursuit of this aim the RATN (Regional AIDS Training Network) was formed. This has been discussed vividly in Chapter 1 wherein are included various facets of RATN like: Formation, Origin and Accomplishments of RATN.

The importance of TRNs (Technical Resource Networks) in the response to HIV/AIDS cannot be left without mention. Chapter 2 defines an agenda for the rapid development of these networks. For the most pact individuals and groups too often work on common problems in isolation from one another. There is a need to make better use of the knowledge of what works against

HIV/AIDS, to increase this knowledge base and to share it more effectively and efficiently. In this context TRNs are becoming increasingly common mechanisms for strengthening and catalysing national responses to HIV/AIDS.

During the mid-1980s, Condom Social Marketing (CSM) emerged as an effective tool in the fight against HIV/AIDS. Through social marketing programmes and projects in many countries affected by the epidemics, condoms have become more easily available, affordable and acceptable to sexually active men, women and young people in general, as well as to those in high risk groups. Chapter 3 discusses six applications of different social marketing techniques drawn from on-going projects in developing countries in the field of reproductive health and prevention of HIV/AIDS and STDs. Individually they illustrate different practical approaches to condom promotion through social marketing in response to particular challenges and needs.

To contain the HIV/AIDS epidemic and reduce its impact we need to expand the response considerably. Chapter 4 proposes a conceptual framework for an expanded response to HIV/AIDS and suggests dimensions along which this response should proceed.

UNAIDS India has through its strategies and programmes, played a critical role in providing a common platform for the UN agencies, the bilaterals, the NGOs and the Government, to work together. Chapter 5 gives an account of the efforts made by UNAIDS India in the year 2000 in enhancing the response to the HIV/AIDS epidemic in India. It addresses the strategies, the interventions and the support structures which have been employed in defining this coordinated and enhanced response.

A discussion of eight selected projects with respect to the UNAIDS Best Practices Criteria (effectiveness, ethical soundness, efficiency, relevance and sustainability) along with a list of issues for consideration of collaborative projects has been undertaken in Chapter 6.

Cost Analysis is a tool that helps in providing useful insight into the functioning of projects as well as being a key component of cost-effectiveness analysis within HIV prevention cost analysis enables managers at project level decide upon the best way to deliver a particular strategy. Chapter 7 to 9 give the importance of Costing Analysis, its fundamentals and choices and a description on planning the costing analysis. A guide to collection and analysis of cost data has been given in Chapter 10.

The principle of greater involvement of people living with or affected by HIV/AIDS (GIPA) was widely acknowledged at the 1994 Paris AIDS Summit but so far precious little has been done towards achieving this aim. Chapter 11 discusses more about GIPA - its meaning, functions, challenges, obstacles, as well as gives suggestions to counter the challenges.

The significant impact of the potential benefits of giving HIV/AIDS a prominent place in PRSPs and HIPC agreements are substantial. Chapters 12 and 13 help enables country officials and their partners prepare and negotiate effectively the inclusion of enhanced HIV/AIDS programmes in the PRSPS (Poverty Reduction Strategy Papers) and instruments of debt relief under the intensified HIPC (Heavily Indebted Poor Country) initiative.

For effective action against AIDS, we need a strong partnership between the public and the private sector. Business should give their expertise and provide financial aid to the national AIDS programme. In return the national AIDS programme should help create a social climate that is conducive to private sector action, an environment that facilitates businesses to participate in AIDS prevention and care. This fact has been brought out clearly in Chapter 14 of this text.

Every year more than one million people emigrate permanently and in most years nearly the same numbers seek asylum. The in-country mobility is far more in numbers. Including both forms of population movement figures of people who move globally each year amount to two billion people. Chapter 15 addresses some of the issues involved in relation to the rights of migrants to health. The study includes arguments related to a number of changes to improve migrants' health (particularly in regard to HIV/AIDS, other sexually transmitted infections and reproductive health) at global national and international levels.

Progress in preventing the spread of HIV/AIDS has been made. The challenge now is to address more comprehensively the complex issues involved, in all countries and at all levels.

One

Development of Regional AIDS Training Network

AIDS has multifarious effects on society. No society has all the requisite skills that will enable it to fight AIDS effectively. The government, organisation or individual involved in HIV/AIDS prevention, care, treatment and support activities needs to have the skills, knowledge and experience to be optimally effective. This can be got through some form of basic or additional training. This training may range from STD control, counselling, testing and community care to behaviour change, managing and planning. Imparting quality education and other training opportunities is the best way of increasing the effectiveness and productivity of management, workers and volunteers on the field. During early 1994, the Universities of Nairobi (Kenya) and Manitoba (Canada) examined the HIV/AIDS related training needs in the Eastern and Southern African (ESA) Region. The study revealed that decision-makers, mid-level managers and trainers throughout the region felt insufficiently prepared to address the growing challenges of HIV/AIDS. While accepting that training was required, the assessment highlighted that training needs differed from country to country.

The Formation of RATN

After assessing the training needs the idea developed to form a network of training institutions and to this effect the Regional AIDS Training Network (RATN) project was founded in 1997. Its object was to impart skills training, upgrading, extension services and technical assistance in the ESA region to health and allied workers in the HIV/AIDS/STDs field.

RATN's aim is to increase the potential of HIV/AIDS/STD programmes there for effective treatment and prevention strategies so as to mitigate the impact of the epidemic.

In its mission, RATN has defined its key functions as:

(a) developing and presenting new training courses through Partner Institutions (PIs) that respond to perceived requirements in the region and

(b) enabling a process that will lead to establishing a formal network of training institutions governed by its members.

Regional AIDS Training Network (RATN) — Origin

The Regional AIDS Training Network began with the long-standing research partnership between the Universities of Nairobi (Kenya) and Manitoba (Canada) in the area of sexually transmitted diseases (STDs). They began working together on STD research and training in the late 1970s. By the early 1980s they had collaborated with the Universities of Washington in the United States and Ghent in Belgium to form the Collaborative Centre for Research and Training in STDs. During the late 1980s, the World Health Organisation (WHO) acclaimed the Centre a "Centre of Excellence" while the Centre accepted WHO's invitation to become a "WHO Collaborating Centre." Other than outstanding work in the natural history and epidemiology of STDs, in 1985 researchers at the Collaborative Centre were the first to discover HIV in Kenya. In times to come, the Collaborative Centre's research and training focus expanded to include the new virus. Further research drew out the now well-established linkages between - STDs and HIV acquisition/transmission, the dynamics of mother-to-child transmission and, lately, proof of a linkage with breast-feeding and the presence in some people of immunity to infection. By the late 1980s and the early 1990s HIV was firmly entrenched and growing in most ESA countries.

The demand for training in STD/HIV prevention, control and treatment at the collaborative centre also grew during this time, with growing demand from all over the region for training opportunities. However, the Collaborating Centre had extremely limited room to keep up with the demand for training. While considering various choices in providing quality STD/HIV training, officials from the Universities of Nairobi and Manitoba, as well as their colleagues from the Centre, pondered over the changing nature of HIV/AIDS in the region and how to solve the spreading epidemic effectively. As the epidemic grew, the multifaceted nature and impact of the virus became increasingly obvious. It became evident that any strategy to prevent the further spread of HIV and to reduce its impact would have to develop beyond the prevention, control and treatment of STDs. This initiated the idea of creating a regional centre to promote excellence in training in a number of areas related to HIV prevention and mitigation of its impact.

To obtain sponsors for a training centre, the universities knew that they had to support their observations on training needs with empirical data. To that effect funds were obtained to carry out a needs assessment study in the ESA region in early 1994. The nine-country study included interviews with major informants and target group discussions with health and allied workers who were considered as potential trainees. The study revealed that decision-makers, mid-level managers and trainers throughout the region were inadequately prepared to address the growing challenges of HIV/AIDS, that training was accepted as a need and that the needs varied from country to country. The study also demonstrated a pattern of isolation with respect to training. Whereas various organisations throughout the regions offered high-quality training courses, many had little knowledge of similar training offered by organisations in other countries. Most institutions offered country-level courses rather than inviting participants from around the region. Furthermore, the study revealed that organisations working in the same field but in different countries did not examine possibilities of sharing training ideas, course content and materials. This was due to deeply held beliefs that countries and institutions in the region had little to learn from each another due to supposed cultural and linguistic differences or variations in local history of the epidemic.

Advantages of the Networking Model

From these conclusions and further discussion in the region originated the idea to form a network of training institutions instead of a training centre. The networking model replaced the concept of the training centre model because it presented some distinct advantages which are given as follows:

(a) Under the training centre model all training would have taken place in one location, while through the networking model, training would take place wherever the training institution was located or needed to provide the course.

(b) Substantial start-up costs were connected with the training centre model including constructing or renting a building(s) to house the training centre, whereas the networking model needed only office space to accommodate a secretariat.

(c) The networking model was considered more economical as the organisations involved would be more prepared to contribute financial and human resources to forming a network in which they had ownership rather than financing a training centre that could be perceived as belonging to somebody else.

The RATN project began in 1997 with the aim of forming a regional network of training institutions to impart skills training, upgrading, extension services and technical help to health and allied workers in the area of HIV/AIDS/STDs in the ESA. RATN's aim is to increase the capacity of HIV/AIDS/STD programmes so as to bring about effective treatment and prevention strategies and, finally, to reduce the epidemic's impact in the region.

Tasks Framed Out by RATN

To achieve its purpose, RATN has designated to itself the following tasks:

(a) identifying and collaborating with high-quality training institutions in ESA to impart regional training courses;

(b) developing and presenting new training courses through PIs in response to understood and felt needs in the region;

(c) providing resources so that existing training programmes can reach a longer spectrum of people;

(d) forming a regional network of technical expertise by convening meetings/work-shops, publishing documents, improving communication linkages, and liasing with institutions and donors;

(e) being a resource for others to identify training institutions, trainers and consultants in the region;
(f) being a focal point for discussions on training issues;
(g) patronising training resources at the regional and international level; and
(h) initiating the establishment of a formal network of training institutions to be administered by its members.

The Training Line

Partner Institutions (PIs) are organisations that have agreed to work with the RATN project on developing and imparting courses as well as forming a formal network of training organisations in the ESA region. There are presently 17 RATN PIs. Together with PIs, RATN has developed courses giving skills training in the following areas: counselling, counselling supervision, syndromic management of STDs, community care of HIV/AIDS, communication and behaviour change, adult education/training of trainers, advocacy, policy and planning of HIV/AIDS, laboratory management, STD supervisor training and adolescent counselling and research. Till now, over 50 training courses have been delivered through RATN PIs, and nearly 700 students from 21 African countries have been trained. RATN courses target not the so-called "front-line workers" but the trainers and managers of programmes.

The idea behind these training of trainers (TOT) courses is that the students will take their newly acquired knowledge and apply it to improving the quality of training given to their own and other institutions as well as individuals keen on training issues in their home countries.

Focus on Network Building

The object of the RATN project then is to build a formal network of organisations involved in training in the HIV/AIDS field. Till now much progress has been made and RATN PIs are generally actively involved in networking (i.e. collaborating, communicating and sharing information).

Accomplishment of RATN

Since its inception, RATN's achievements have been notable. They include:

(i) High degree of satisfaction with RATN courses

The follow-up studies of RATN course alumni show that the alumni and their employing organisation are highly content with the courses. One alumni follow-up study from the counselling and community care courses offered by RATN and its PIs demonstrate that over 80 per cent of the respondents bettered their operational skills in the workplace, and a large percentage commented on increased levels of faith and interpersonal skills and clients.

(ii) Increasing the standard of training in the region

RATN has started to have a major impact on raising the standard for training in the ESA region. The use of expert committees to define minimal and optimal training constituents of new RATN courses has enabled them gain a reputation for setting new, improved training standards.

(iii) Demonstrating the value of training

RATN and its PIs are working together to raise awareness among decision-makers and donors of the importance of quality training. Using the results of its monitoring and evaluation activities, RATN can demonstrate the short and long-term results and advantage of its courses.

(iv) Bridging the Communication Gap between Partner Institutions (PIs)

RATN has had some accomplishment in breaking the relative isolation that exists in the ESA region among training organisations in the HIV/AIDS field, specially those offering training in counselling and community care.

Challenges Faced by RATN

RATN and its PIs have faced several challenges in working toward their goals. They include the following:

(A) Challenges faced during course delivery

(i) *Choosing the course participants:* RATN and the PIs have carefully defined admission needs for each course and closely examined course application forms. Even then, some alumni are not satisfied with the level of knowledge of other course participants and the negative effect this had had on their learning experience.

(ii) *Financing the course participants:* Some funders have criticized RATN for utilizing operational funds to directly support scholarships for course participants. RATN accepts that in under ideal circumstances it would not have to do so. However, the status of regional economics—course delivery costs as well as the inability of most individuals and AIDS service organisations to bear the costs for training—mean that RATN must underwrite a certain amount of training costs at least for the time being.

(iii) *Follow up Post course:* RATN alumni have signalled the need for post-course support and follow-up to help them fully take advantage of the knowledge they have gained. RATN and its PIs are currently evaluating cost-effective strategies to respond to this expressed requirement.

(B) Challenges Faced during Network-Building

While much advances have been made in establishing a formal network the RATN PIs are, to varying degrees, actively occupied in the process of networking. Many project sponsors expected that more progress would have been made by now. To address this challenge, a network development committee has been given a formal go ahead to explore options for establishing a formal network, a governance structure for the network, and a time-frame for setting up the network as a distinct legal entity.

(C) Promoting Collaboration between Partner Institutions (PIs)

RATN has found some success in promoting collaboration between its PIs, particularly between those PIs that are offering courses in the same field (i.e. counselling and community care). However, it has been less successful in encouraging collaboration between PIs that offer courses in disparate areas.

(D) Funding

Funding has been RATN's major challenges. There are two aspects to this concern. The first involves reaching out adequate resources to cover RATN's planned activities and the second further expand its funding base.

Lessons Learned

Since its beginning, the RATN project has undertaken a number of lessons learned exercises.

Lessons learned about training

1. *Conducting a needs assessment study:* This is an important initial step in implementing intervention programmes. Using needs assessment data in programme planning helps ensure that interventions are according to actual needs. Such programmes are likely to attract support from different sponsors. The needs assessment study that was conducted prior to the RATN project's development obtained information that helped ensure that the project was relevant to needs of the ESA region, and has contributed to RATN's success at fund-raising.
2. *Developing an ongoing resource for identifying emerging needs:* This is a way of maintaining context compliance. Expert committees have been valuable to ensuring that the RATN courses are relevant and have also helped in raising the standard for training in the ESA region.
3. *RATN courses have been adapted to suit the needs of the ESA region:* This has contributed to making them relevant and popular. This practice has significantly decreased the number of courses that are not relevant, hitherto a common phenomena, especially with courses from the first world countries.
4. *Creating and initiating a culture of excellence in course content and delivery among PIs:* This has made a substantial impact in several areas. It has increased awareness of the need for quality training: created a demand for the courses being offered and swiftly made RATN and its partners acclaimed regional advisers on best practices in training.
5. *Giving feedback of results into programmes:* The practice of feeding back the results of monitoring and evaluation exercises into programmes and activities guarantees constant quality control and improvement of courses and training.
6. *Follow-up studies are important:* They measure the impact of training on alumni and their employing organisations.

The data from the studies helps analyse the course's impact and this information can be used to improve subsequent programmes. Such data also measure the effectiveness of the training offered.

Lessons learned about collaborating and networking

1. *PIs (members) are more expected to contribute to developing a network if the contribution of their participation is clear:* It is important to create continuous opportunities for PIs to reflect on how their organisations are benefiting from their involvement to keep them motivated.
2. *It is important for PIs in a network to have direct contact with one another:* At the same time they should not to become overly reliant on secretariat staff to enable communications.
3. *Giving a sense of Project Ownership:* Their participation in the governance of the RATN project has given PIs a sense of project ownership and increased their motivation to achieving a formal network of training institutions.
4. *Formalise through resources and planning:* Building a formal network will not be achieved just by being involved in networking activities like information-sharing and promoting collaboration. Such activities are important in creating a feel of working for a common goal but they will not in themselves give members a feeling that the network belongs to the. Building a formal network needs resources and a solid plan as to how to establish and sustain it.
5. *Need for communication channels:* Directing funds in communication channels such as the RATN member newsletter and the RATN web site has been a powerful way to keep PIs informed of important information and resources. They have also helped to improve the public image of RATN and PI projects along with that of their courses, throughout the ESA region.

Need for Training

Imparting of high-quality courses and other training opportunities is a well tested means of increasing the effectiveness and productivity of management, workers and volunteers in the workplace. The effect of HIV/AIDS on any given sector of society and the economy are multiple and complex. All organisations and individuals engaged in HIV/AIDS prevention, care, treatment and support activities can take advantage from basic or additional training, whether it be STD control, counselling and testing, community care, behaviour change, or managing and planning. In the challenging field of HIV/AIDS work new developments are constantly taking place. Keeping up with these developments is vital. Training makes sure that individuals and organisations in a wide spectrum of areas stay informed of new developments, new techniques and approaches, recognized good practices and how to use them effectively. Almost 20 years of living with the HIV virus has also earmarked that the tension of working in the HIV/AIDS field can lead to high rates of turnover and exhaustion. When people leave government or other organisations working in HIV/AIDS, or shift jobs, training is required to give new people the skills and confidence to perform well at their jobs and to help keep the organisations with whom they work effective, innovative and committed. Sending employees on training courses to upgrade their knowledge and skills is also a well tested antidote against burnout. One important factor leading to burnout is the concern at being ill-equipped to perform responsibilities as well as expected. In many examples employees or volunteers lack the expertise and skills to meet performance expectations but quality training helps them to work more effectively in many situations and can relieve them of this stress.

Key Functions of RATN

(I) RATN: Management and Staff Overview

The RATN project is managed by a secretariat located on the grounds of the College of Health Sciences at the University of Nairobi in Kenya. The secretariat mainly helps in the development of the project's work plan and its effective implementation. The project staff includes two co-directors, a project manager, two programme coordinators and a few support staff:

The co-directors: represent the two main project partners - the Universities of Nairobi and Manitoba. They serve as the project's senior managers and together are responsible for overall project operations. There duties include: strategic planning; project monitoring and evaluation; fund-raising; liaison with and reporting to donors and the Kenyan Ministry of Health; and maintaining links with PIs and other leading regional and international HIV/ AIDS organisations.

The project manager: is incharge of for project administration, financial management and reporting, and human resource management.

The course coordinator: has overall charge for developing and delivering courses. This includes liasing with PIs to develop, schedule, monitor and evaluate courses, organize expert committee meetings and follow up with course alumni.

The network coordinator: is incharge of initiating a formal network of training institutions and provides services to RATN members. This comprises: supporting the Network Development Committee, marketing courses, developing the RATN web site, producing and distributing the RATN newsletter, and liasing and maintaining communication with other regional AIDS and STD networks.

The RATN co-directors, project manager and programme coordinators are backed up by a small number of full and part-time staff, consisting of resources centre librarian, a data entry clerk and an information officer. Together with these the secretariat employs consultants on an as-needed basis for special assignments.

(II) RATN and PIs Collaborations

The RATN secretariat's collaborative role with the PIs includes cooperation in the following key areas:

(a) course development
(b) course delivery
(c) monitoring and evaluation
(d) long-term follow-up
(e) network building

This collaboration is addressed more clearly in the section on the key activities of RATN (see ahead in this chapter). The RATN secretariat and PIs also collaborate in project planning, workshops, advocacy and course marketing described as follows:

(i) Project Planning

In collaboration with PIs the RATN secretariat evolves an annual action plan to achieve the project's goal and objectives. The secretariat demands that PIs make comments and suggestions during the planning process. The steering committee, which has representatives from the PIs as well as the Universities of Nairobi and Manitoba, donors, and other interested parties, adopts the final work plan.

(ii) Workshops

Sometimes the RATN Secretariat and the PIs work together on developing and implementing workshops to advance RATN's work. Workshops on monitoring and evaluation, advocacy and marketing have been arranged to develop strategies for implementation by both the secretariat and the PIs, and other PI workshops are worked out on specific areas of interest.

(iii) Advocacy

RATN and the PIs are committed to raising awareness of the need for and the availability of quality training in the region. This concern for advocacy as collaborative effort is explained more specifically in the section of RATN and the promotion of training (see below).

(iv) Course marketing

The RATN secretariat and PIs both play a role in marketing RATN affiliated courses. The secretariat produces a course calendar and distributes it to a mailing list of potential clients and donors; the calendar is also posted on the RATN web site and updated in the quarterly newsletter. PIs receive the RATN newsletter for distribution and also promote RATN courses in their respective newsletters.

Collaboration with RATN - the Partner's Experience

When questioned as to why they value their participation in RATN, PIs responded:

RATN has helped us raise our image as a training organisation. We have benefitted from our collaboration with

RATN in many ways. RATN has, for example, provided us with an opportunity to share and review course, curricula and exchange information and materials with RATN and other PIs around the region.

Through RATN, my organisation has had the qualitative aspects of its courses examined by other PIs and the RATN Secretariat. This free of charge 'peer review' has resulted in better quality, delivery and effectiveness/relevance of our courses.

I find the information contained on the RATN web site to be very useful, in especially the workshop reports and the training information. RATN has provided us many more opportunities to share information and interact with other institutions than we had before joining. The partnership has enabled the programme to dwell into new [training] areas that we had not thought of offering at a regional level. Staff members have been trained in various courses through RATN... this has improved our service delivery in the communities we are serving. Exposure to other environments has helped to examine some of our systems [and] our monitoring skills have been enhanced.

My organisation gets a lot of benefit from its participation in RATN, including the marketing of our courses, staff development, friendship and networking with others in the region. Our participation in RATN gives us a regional-as opposed to local-perspective of what is happening to fight AIDS.

RATN Partner Institutions (PIs)

The organisations working with the RATN project on developing and providing courses and creating a formal network of training organisations in ESA are known as Partner Institutions (PIs). There are currently 17 RATN PIs:

(i) Centre for African Studies (CAFS), Nairobi, Kenya
(ii) Connect Institute of Systemic Therapy, Harare, Zimbabwe
(iii) Eastern and Southern Africa Management Institute (ESAMI), Arusha, United Republic of Tanzania
(iv) Family Aids Caring Trust (FACT), Mutare, Zimbabwe
(v) Genitourinary Centre, Harare, Zimbabwe
(vi) Health Economics and HIV/AIDS Research Division (HEARD), University of Natal. Durban, South Africa

(vii) KARA Counselling and Training Trust Limited, Lusaka, Zambia

(viii) Kenyan Association of Professional Counsellors (KAPC), Nairobi, Kenya

(ix) Malawi Institute of Management (MIM), Lilongwe, Malawi

(x) Mildmay International, Kampala, Uganda

(xi) Project Support Group, University of Zimbabwe, Harare, Zimbabwe

(xii) Salvation Army Chikankata Health Services, Chikankata, Zambia

(xiii) School of Public Health, Nelson Mandela College of Medicine, University of Natal, South Africa

(xiv) South Africa Institute for Medical Research (SAIMR), Johannesburg, South Africa

(xv) The AIDS Service Organisation (TASO), Kampala, Uganda

(xvi) The United Republic of Tanzania Gender Network Programme (TGNP), Dar es Salaam, United Republic of Tanzania

(xvii) University of Nairobi, Kenya

(III) RATN and the Promotion of Quality Training

One of RATN's main roles is to improve the variety and quality of training in the region. This helps people to address the threat of the HIV/AIDS epidemic. The most obvious way that RATN tries to achieve this is by collaborating with PIs to develop, deliver and improve the quality of training courses. A less obvious way in which RATN and its PIs perform this role is through advocacy. For organisations and individuals in the front lines of the reaction to the epidemic the need for effective training is clear. However, in the experience of RATN and its PIs the need to invest in training is still undermined by most decision-makers.

The 1994 training needs assessment study found out significant gaps between the stated need for training in certain areas and available courses. The long-term follow-up and evaluation of course alumni and their supervisors from counselling and community care of HIV/AIDS courses revealed that many decision-makers do not give much thought to the quality, efficiency or utility of the available training as long as it takes place.

For instance, the examination found that many decision-makers made hardly any effort to discuss with trainees the quality of the training received or to find out from them the impact and implications of their new knowledge and skills for the individual or the organisation. More so, many decision-makers did not give the necessary support for trainees to utilize their new knowledge and skills, which is important if training is to make a difference.

Training Champions

If individuals in a position to provide resources for HIV/AIDS do not understand the need for quality training and for ensuring that the trainees' acquisition of new knowledge and skills is supported, then training requires a champion.

Since the beginning the RATN project and its PIs have taken on this role with some notable achievements. Representatives from RATN have been invited to meetings on behalf of the training sector and the RATN model has been referred to in major policy documents as an example that should and could be followed in other regions. Given the importance of raising the profile of training in the ESA region, RATN and its PIs will continue to devote time and resources to advocating for the cause of training. They are currently examining the best strategies for achieving this.

(IV) Information dissemination

Another key function of the RATN secretariat is to compile and disseminate information compliant to the needs of the PIs and the RATN project itself. RATN accomplishes this by-producing a newsletter, supporting a web site, creating marketing courses, developing and maintaining a resource centre and enabling electronic networking between PIs.

RATN Newsletter and website

The quarterly RATN newsletter gives information on RATN committee meetings, workshops, events, member news and other developments in HIV/AIDS-related training. The newsletter is distributed to over 2000 readers consisting of PIs, course alumni, donors, potential trainees and course sponsors, which includes government department, local and international nongovernmental organisations (NGOs), and multilateral organisations throughout the region. The RATN web site - www.ratn.org contains information regarding course as well as database and newsletter can be scanned through it.

Resource Centre

The RATN secretariat accommodates a small resource centre focusing on subjects related to the prevention, care, treatment and support of HIV/AIDS, training and evaluation. Members may borrow from the centre's collection and are kept informed of latest developments.

Electronic Networking

The RATN secretariat encourages the use of electronic mail to PIs as a way of communicating with the secretariat and one another. It also promotes the use of Internet to access information and resources related to HIV/AIDS and/or training among the PIs. The secretariat is presently seeking funds to ensure access to electronic mail and the Internet for all PIs. There has been rapid progress in telecommunications capabilities in the region in the few years since RATN was founded, and it continues to monitor recent developments so that the recent technological changes can be utilized to maintain and improve communications between PIs and with the secretariat.

Activities of RATN

(I) Designing Courses

One of RATN's main activities is to identify and establish linkages with training institutions and through them to design, develop and deliver short courses aimed at middle-level workers, managers and trainers in the ESA region. Together with the PIs, RATN it has created courses providing skills training in the following areas:

> Counselling, counselling supervision, syndromic management of STDs, community care of HIV/AIDS, communication and behaviour change, adult education/training of trainers, advocacy, policy & planning of HIV/AIDS, laboratory management, STD supervisor training and adolescent counselling & research.

RATN courses are designed for trainers and programme managers. Training of trainers (TOT) courses are developed on the idea that the students will take their new-found knowledge and apply it for improving the quality of training given by their own and other institutions in their parent countries.

(II) Expert Committees for Training Development

Building of excellence is a core principle underlying RATN's philosophy of course development. To further this, RATN has evolved a process that involves the use of expert committees. For most new courses offered under the patronage of RATN, the course coordinator convenes an expert committee. This is done by canvassing PIs, donors and other chosen individuals and organisations/institutions to identify individuals acknowledged for their knowledge, skills and experience in a given subject area as well as trainers known for their exceptional skills and experience.

Nominees receive a letter presenting the committee's terms of reference (TORs) and inviting them to attend a three- to five-day meeting, which generally takes the form of a facilitator-led workshop. The TORs of any given expert committee typically include the following:

(a) Recognition of the optimal components of a training programme, including modules on TOT or managerial courses that need to be included to the basic curriculum.
(b) Develop the minimum standard for an acceptable course curriculum.
(c) Identify training institutions in the region that are holding high-quality training courses related to HIV/AIDS.
(d) Identify lacunal in existing courses and suggest ways to enhance them.
(e) Identify courses that are required but not currently offered.

The first meeting of any expert committee tackles at least the first three or four of these TORs. In most cases courses are offered by at least one or two institutions within a year of the meeting. Expert committee follow-up meetings are usually held every two years to monitor courses, paying particular attention to the student evaluations collected. Suggestions are made to the training institutions on improvements to modify their courses. Committee members also identify emerging trends and new issues, and suggest how they might influence course content, recommend improvements to courses and select new courses that need to be developed.

In the same way the Community Care of HIV Expert Committee meeting in October 1997 identified a training syllabus. This course is now delivered by three PIs in the region: TASO (Uganda), Salvation Army Chikankata (Zambia) and FACT (Zimbabwe). A follow-up meeting in October 1999 examined these courses, and new course areas were proposed for development. The community care group met again in September 2000 to develop these courses further, more so in the areas of caring for the carers and palliative care.

A course of palliative care was held in Uganda in 2001.

Expert Committees in Action

The first expert committee meeting in counselling was held in March 1997. The meeting identified a training syllabus for a counselling TOT course, and three institutions (Kenyan Association of Professional Counsellors (KAPC) Nairobi, KARA Counselling and Training Trust Limited, Lusaka, and Connect Institute of Systemic Therapy, Harare) subsequently began to deliver this course. A follow-up counselling meeting in April 1999 reviewed these courses and recommended new counselling courses. Consequently, "Counselling supervisor training" and "Counselling adolescents" courses were launched in 2000.

(III) Course Delivery

Since KAPC arranged the first RATN-sponsored course in late 1997, more than 50 training courses have been held through PIs, and almost 700 students from 21 African countries have been trained. RATN courses are held in locations all over the ESA region, primarily in the city, town or rural location of the PI that is giving the course. Most courses are residential, and the fees is inclusive of room and board costs. The courses are of two to five weeks' duration. RATN courses mainly employ local trainers affiliated with the PI, although in some cases trainers from other institutions or from outside the ESA region are utilized. From the outset RATN has been aware of the need to ensure a gender balance among course participants. To date there has been a balance between number of women and men attending RATN courses, with women predominating slightly. Similarly, RATN consciously tries to ensure that students chosen to attend the courses come from as many of the countries in the ESA region as possible. All RATN courses offered have had students from a minimum of three ESA countries. The RATN secretariat and the PIs work closely together examining the application forms for each course, so as to achieve a balance of genders, skills and regional representation from the number of available applicants.

(IV) Post Course Evaluation

Advantages

From the very start, RATN recognized that the key to its success and the skill to recognise success when it happened, was in developing a firm and detailed system of monitoring and evaluation. To evaluate courses, each RATN course participant fills up a standardised evaluation form at the end of his or her course. Student evaluations are compared carefully and shared with the PI responsible for the course so it can make any necessary changes in the content or training methods. The evaluation results may also be used as resource materials by the expert committees. Their utility is particularly clear when more than one RATN PI offers similar courses at different times. The post-course evaluation data allow for a comparative analysis between the courses offered by the different PIs. The comparative analysis results are shared with each of the PIs and expert committees, who use them to modify course content and training methods.

A RATN evaluation performed in the fall of 1999 by the Canadian International Development Agency quoted RATN's practice of performing a comparative analysis of post-course evaluation data from similar courses as "an innovative way" to monitor and control the quality and content of training courses.

(V) Long term Follow up and Evaluation of RATN

RATN carried out a follow-up study of course alumni and their supervisors from counselling and community care of HIV/ AIDS courses. During 2000, with funding from UNAIDS and cooperation with the PIs. The study examined whether the courses have had any impact or influence on: (a) the participant and his/her professional skills; and (b) on the employing organisation and the community. The evaluation exercise was also utilized to share the results with others wanting to learn from the RATN model. The study methodology, findings and impact of the findings on RATN are as follows:

Study Methodology and Tools

A convenience sample was used in this study. The focus was on the alumni who completed their course at least six months previously and their supervisors. The study sought to interview all available alumni and their supervisors and to conduct focus group discussions with traceable alumni. A total of 90 alumni and 74 of their supervisors from 5 countries (Kenya, Malawi, Uganda, Zambia and Zimbabwe) were interviewed. These 90 alumni included a 61.2 per cent rate out of the possible total (ranging from 85.2 per cent follow-up rate in Uganda to 37.9 per cent in Zimbabwe). The alumni were employed by a variety of organisations, including government institutions, NGOs and universities. Among the respondents, 71 per cent came from capital cities while 29 per cent were from other smaller towns. Major findings of the study are presented as follows:

Impact on the Course Participants

Cited relevance of courses

(a) Alumni felt that the skills they learned in the course were in context to their current job. Over 62 per cent reported transferability of skills to their work environment as the most useful course attribute.
(b) A large percentage of participating alumni from both the counselling and community care courses felt increased levels of confidence and interpersonal skills with clients.

Increased skills

(a) Over 81 per cent of the alumni reported having improved their operational skills in the work place. Counselling alumni reported increased counselling skills and community care alumni reported enhanced provision of community care services.

(b) Thirty-six percent of the alumni felt that their job responsibilities changed as a result of course participation. Those alumni whose responsibilities shifted indicated that additional duties were assigned or duties shifted because the course had enhanced their knowledge and skills and they were more competent in handling certain issues, especially those related to HIV/AIDS. At times even, job responsibilities changed because the course participant initiated new programmed after attending the training course.

(VI) Impact on the Employing Organisation and the Community

Influence on peers

(a) The majority of alumni (97.8 per cent) reported having shared the course experience with members of their organisation. The information was shared with the immediate supervisor in 78 per cent of cases; with colleagues in 91.2 per cent and less frequently with policy-makers/planners.

(b) As alumni went back to their jobs and communities, they shared the knowledge they acquired during the course. Of the alumni, 45.1 per cent reported used the knowledge and skills from the course to develop in-service training programmes, to organise formal training programmes (35.2 per cent) and to influence policy formulation (27.5 per cent).

Influence on the Organisation Employing the Alumni

(a) Supervisors of course alumni felt that courses offered very contextual training that benefitted their organisation and identified a range of benefits, including improved services to clients, initiation of new client services, strengthened staff capacity, improved monitoring and evaluation, and better fund utilization.

(b) Some target group discussion participants stated that their organisations received recognition and legitimization due to improved community services provided by trained alumni.

Strengthened networking among participants

(a) RATN courses play a crucial role in strengthening networking among course attendants. Over 85 per cent of alumni indicated that they have been sharing information with fellow participants and 78 per cent were communicating with others working in similar fields.

(b) Target group discussions clearly point out that greater and stronger collaboration between organisations developed as a result of individual connections established during the training courses. One participant reported the effect thus: We have broadened our collaboration and networking and we no longer work in isolation."

(c) At the organisational level, networking or increased collaboration has resulted in exchanging information and course materials, holding joint seminars, exchanging course facilitators, inviting guest speakers to forums, and organising formal and informal meetings.

The Need for Post Training Follow-up

Results from focus group discussions and the survey show that alumni require support from their colleagues, supervisors, planners and policy-makers to make the optimum use of the skills gained during training. Alumni indicated feeling constrained by the lack of follow-up support for further collaboration, learning, and supervision after completing RATN training courses. Alumni wanted follow-up meetings where they could "share experiences" and "seek help when problems arise."

Impact on RATN Development

The study findings have had a major impact on RATN's development and future direction. The findings indicate that the training courses in counselling and community care have brought about positive results for the alumni and the organisations with whom they work, and prefer that the clients and communities served by course alumni also benefit from the alumni's enhanced performance. These results are crucial in themselves because in a "results-oriented" funding atmosphere they represent measurable "outcomes", which are important to demonstrating to donors and their constituencies the effectiveness of training. Moreover, these results will be an effective tool when RATN and its PIs advocate on behalf of training in the region. Whereas the follow-up study results have strengthened RATN's and the PIs' recognition for measuring the impact of training courses this also presents a clear challenge.

Follow up studies are costly and time-consuming for the PIs and the RATN secretariat. Financial and human resources are hard to find for such studies. Undertaking additional follow-up studies means that RATN and the PIs will have to divert funds currently meant for course development and course delivery or raise additional funds. Whereas, the existing follow-up study methodology could be improved to make it more cost-effective and time-efficient for RATN secretariat staff and the PIs.

RATN and the PIs are presently involved in examining all of the options for future monitoring and evaluation activities, including follow-up studies.

Impact of Counselling and Community Care Courses

(i) The relevance of knowledge and skills delivered through the training courses is necessary for their application at the organisational level. Transferability of skills to work situations was reported by 62.3 per cent of the alumni as the most useful course attribute.

(ii) A prime feature of the collaboration in the regional courses is to assist participants in improving skills that may lead to improved quality of serviçes. Over 81 per cent of respondents reported that the courses helped them to modify their operational skills in the workplace.

(iii) For the impact of training to be felt at the organisational level, dissemination of the course outcome by the alumni within their organisation must take place. Supervisors confirmed that over 90 per cent of those attended RATN courses had shared knowledge and skills gained from the course within the organisation.

(iv) Supervisors recognised the advantage of the training to their organisations. Over 87 per cent indicated that the training has improved service to clients and over 83 per cent noted that it strengthened the capacity of their organisation's staff.

(v) Participation in RATN courses improved networking among course alumni. Over 87 per cent of alumni report that they made new contact as a result of the course they attended.

(vi) Alumni report the need for some form of post-training support so as to ensure that they are able to fully apply the skills and knowledge they learned during the course.

Building the RATN Network

As has been discussed earlier RATN is as much about network building as about course delivery. Off late the RATN secretariat and PIs have taken numerous steps to establish a formal network. Major milestones in the network's history are:

(a) employing a network coordinator in the RATN secretariat;
(b) drafting the network strategy paper;
(c) enabling meetings and opportunities for PIs, donors and other key stakeholders to reflect on the draft networking strategy and other aspects of network development;
(d) arranging for a legal opinion on the network's options for its structure and incorporation;
(e) developing up a network development committee and giving it a mandate to propose strategies for a sustainable, self-governing network and
(f) informing donors and potential donors of the want to formalize the network

Even though a formal network has yet to be achieved, it is improper to conclude that RATN PIs have not realized the benefits of "networking" or do not feel part of a network. Although a formal network was not established when the Canadian International Development Agency (CIDA) conducted its 1999 mid-project review, PIs indicated feeling part of a regional network in which they could make contacts with colleagues in other countries. They also indicated benefits to their programmes as a result of collaborating through RATN. For PIs, the networking benefits are most obvious among those institutions that offer courses in the same subject area. For instance, the CIDA evaluation documented that three PIs initially thought themselves to be competitors because each offers counselling courses, but they now frequently communicate about course content and training, and have attended each other's courses. Infact, these three institutions are now looking at collaborating to develop and deliver courses.

Further proof of RATN's networking impact and added value in the region comes from the professional associations and sub-networks that it has helped initiate. Malawian alumni from various RATN counselling courses formed the Malawian Association of Counsellors. Similarly, RATN alumni and counselling PIs also spawned the East and Southern Africa Counselling Association (ESACA). Each of these associations has successfully obtained funding from donors who were partly motivated by their alliance with RATN. During 1999, UNAIDS requested and funded RATN to help set up an independent network of organisations involved in delivering community care services — the Community Care Resource Network (CCN). A CCN interim steering committee, including NGO representatives and RATN PIs, has been established and a short-term plan has been made for the network's development. RATN has been given a mandate to hire, assist and supervise the network coordinator. RATN's support role in CCN's development is expected to progress as the network matures.

Two

Technical Resource Networks

TRNs in Response to HIV/AIDS

What are TRNs?

An attempt has been made in the study to examine the importance of TRNs (Technical Resource Networks) in response to HIV/AIDS. TRNs are becoming increasingly common mechanising for strengthening and catalysing national response to AIDS/HIV.

Definitions

Technical Resource Networks are groups of individuals coming from communities, private institutions and governments that work together towards a shared objective: to help achieve specified goals and to improve the performance of programmes supported by network members. Networks can operate at global, regional or national levels. The term 'network' has largely been used to describe a range of coalitions and organisations, which work together in the field of HIV/AIDS. These networks can vary from specialized 'think tanks' on different aspects of the epidemic to regional support networks, linking together people and programmes with shared challenges. Networking includes making contacts and encouraging reciprocal information exchange, meetings and voluntary collaboration. Networking should initiate and facilitate the autonomy of colleagues rather than reinforcing dependency associations (Starkey, 1997).

Characteristics of Technical Resource Networks

(a) Common goals and interests
(b) Members (individuals, projects, programmes, research institutions)
(c) Regular communications

(d) Focus on a specific issue and/or region
(e) Coordinating mechanism (secretariat, managing committee)
(f) Common workplan and operational budget

Types of Technical Resource Networks

TRNs exist in various forms and for several purposes. For example, a network can focus on a particular theme and particular geographic region, such as the newiy formed AIDS Strategic Planning Network in Western and Central Africa. Networks may be classified according to their geographic scope, thematic focus or membership criteria.

Geographic scope: Networks may be at the global, regional, national or sub-national level. During 1999, the UNAIDS Secretariat reviewed a convenience sample of 52 networks being supported UNAIDS (UNAIDS 1999). The results showed that 23 networks (44.2 per cent) were at the global level; 25 networks (48.1 per cent) at the regional level; 3 networks (5.8 per cent) at the sub-regional level; and 1 network (1.9 per cent) at the country level.

Thematic networks: These specifically address a single subject or group of subjects. They may among the basic disciplines that underpin responses to HIV/AIDS - for instance, the International AIDS Economics Network and the Reference Group on Estimates and Modelling of HIV/AIDS. Others comprise networks of persons working on the prevention of Mother-to-Child Transmission of HIV and networks on how to access pharmaceuticals. Some TRNs emphasize on developing practical skills and/or building competencies in specific disciplines. Examples include the Africa-based Regional AIDS Training Network and the Asian Harm Reduction Network. Some networks were set up primarily to exchange the latest research methods and findings in HIV/AIDS. These networks include the Reference Group on Estimates and Modelling of HIV/AIDS. Monitoring the AIDS Pandemic Network, and HIV Virus Isolation and Characterization Network. Six of the networks sampled by UNAIDS symbolize inter-agency working groups with varying frequencies of meetings and intensity of activities.

Membership: Some networks are closed while others are open. Closed networks tend to emphasize on technical subjects of interest to a small number of specialists. An example of a closed network is the Reference Group on Estimates and Modelling of HIV/AIDS. Open networks are less specialized. An example of an open network is SAFCO, an independent public forum on the response to HIV/AIDS in French-speaking Western and Central Africa. Individuals wishing to join SAFCO may do so by accessing the website "http://www.hivnet.ch/fdp/".

Line of Action in Networking

Due to the complex nature of the HIV/AIDS epidemic and the varying capacities of countries and institutions to respond to it, there are wide differences in the scope, effectiveness and efficiency of responses to HIV/AIDS. From experiences from around the world, effective approaches, policies, strategies and technologies are identified as 'best practice' by the UNAIDS Secretariat and Co-sponsors. The attitude of best practice goes beyond documentation: practices and lessons learned are promoted and disseminated through the UNAIDS Best Practice Collection, pilot projects, country-level programmes, technical assistance, exchange forums and technical resource networks. TRNs help to modify availability of, and accessibility to, technical know-how. This is needed to help countries and local groups in their response to the HIV epidemic. The following are the rationale around which networking is built:

(a) The most important rationale for networking is to improve the impact of programmes in response to HIV/AIDS, measured in terms of tangible reductions in the incidence of HIV, adequate care for persons living with HIV/AIDS and the reduction of impacts on individuals, households and countries.

(b) By developing capacity, improving knowledge, providing technical support and sharing approaches and best practices, the networks have both improved on HIV prevention efforts on the ground and influenced policy development at the regional and national levels.

The speeding up of national-level efforts to expand the response the HIV/AIDS epidemic has resulted in a phenomenal rise in demand for technical resources - both information and expertise - in a widening range of programme areas. At the same time, effective programme strategies are often specific to cultural, resource and political environments. Individual agencies have made, and continue to make, large contributions in specific areas of HIV prevention and care. But it is also largely evident that single institutions, whether government departments, UN agencies, non-governmental organisations (NGOs), or groups of people living with HIV/AIDS, do not have the strength to deal with the multiple determinants of HIV on their own. The need to act simultaneously and synergistically in a number of areas such as well focused interventions, health services, communications, legal reform, education, rural development and the status of women, needs that a range of technical issues must be addressed at the same time. This has further enhanced the need within countries for access to current technical information and expertise.

Factors Influencing Performance Levels in HIV/AIDS Control

The major factors influencing the level of performance include the following:

(a) The policy background, including demonstrated political commitment by government and the commitment of the civil society.
(b) Strength-technical, managerial and political - to analyse problems and to develop effective strategies for tackling them
(c) Transparency of objectives in specific and measurable terms
(d) Information (and knowledge) base
(e) Utilizing scientific evidence of what works in the response to HIV/AIDS.
(f) Quality, compliance and timeliness of inputs
(g) Financial and human resources
(h) Technology as a means of exchange of information and knowledge
(i) Harmony between interventions and institutions with responsibility for implementing them.

Networks can help to strengthen the response to HIV/AIDS by modifying the quality of technical support in each of these areas.

What do TRNs Help to Achieve

Key Functions

Networks help in building local technical capacity, national and regional advocacy, sharing of information, peer support and aiding collective action. They create influential coalitions among programmes, giving them the crucial mass needed to respond to HIV/AIDS at the global, regional and national levels. At the regional level, they help to solve cross-border issues that may drive or be the result of the HIV/AIDS epidemic and at the local level, networks can be highly successful in sharing skills, information, resources and peer support. The TRNs broadly contribute in the following aspects of AIDS/HIV programmes:

Functions of TRNs

(A) Capacity Building

(i) Acting as a resource on different areas of responses to HIV/AIDS.

(ii) Strengthening the potential of local communities and programmes to respond to HIV/AIDS, thus reducing reliance on outside assistance.

(iii) Sharing global and regional expertise with partners at the country level

(B) Solidarity and Advocacy

(i) Reducing isolation of members and giving support;

(ii) Strengthening responses in important but poorly implemented areas of HIV/AIDS.;

(C) Information Sharing

(i) Initiating the exchange of ideas, understanding, experience and skills

(ii) Exchanging and documenting best strategies from global, regional and national experience.

(D) Funding

(i) Mobilizing and Utilizing Financial AID for Optimum Results

Most importantly, networks can actually enable the development of new programmes and policies. Thereby helping to reduce a region's reliance on direct external assistance. This, in turn, builds capacity and enlarges the network's functioning. A single network may not perform all the functions outlines above, several TRNs based at the Institute Nacional de Salud Publica in Cuernavaca, Mexico perform most of these key functions, described in the following paragraph.

TRNs based at the Instituto Nacional de Salud Publica, Cuernavaca, Mexico

This UNAIDS Collaborating Centre has a large range of activities AIDS education and research. In addition, it serves as the headquarters for the following networks:

(a) *Latin American Network on Women and AIDS (Glams):* This network facilitates research and prevention of HIV infection among women in Latin America with the help of an information exchange network and advocacy. Its programmes include development and distribution of a quarterly newsletter; maintenance of a website and an electronic discussion forum; and publications on AIDS and women in Latin America. It receives financial aid from the MacArthur Foundation.

(b) *AIDS and Economics in Latin America (SEAL):* This network promotes communication among researchers working on AIDS and economics in Latin America. It modifies access to information on research related to the economic determinants and impact of AIDS in Latin America. Its activities include maintenance of a website and an electronic discussion forum; technical publications; maintenance of a virtual library of grey literature on AIDS and economics in Latin America; and development of methods for National AIDS Accounts. It collaborates with and/or receives financial aid from SIDALAC, UNAIDS and IAEN.

(c) *Latin American Network on AIDS and Strategic Planning (REDPES):* This network aims at: (a) promoting communication among researchers and policy-makers working on AIDS and strategic planning in Latin America and (b) modifying access to information and strengthen capacity for strategic planning on AIDS. Its activities include — (a) provision of technical assistance on strategic planning and AIDS, (b) exchange of experiences with other regional networks; and (c) maintenance of a website and an electronic discussion forum. It collaborates with and is financed by UNAIDS. REDPES is of the view that strategic plans should be considered as guiding documents that are open to adjustment. Such plans have either been completed or are in draft forms is several countries in the region. In six countries (Chile, Peru, Colombia, Guatemala, Honduras and Mexico) REDPES has promoted the development of "integrated plans" for United Nations agencies in the Thematic Groups that aid the national strategic plans.

In the 1999 review of TRNs cited earlier, UNAIDS Secretariat staff members were asked to identify the overall objectives of the networks with which they collaborated. More than one objective was marked where appropriate. The following objectives have been identified as percentages in the different networks:

(a) exchange of information, experience, or scientific findings;
(b) advocacy;
(c) support to strategy development;
(d) capacity building through workshops or meetings;
(e) resource mobilization; and
(f) other.

Figures indicate that the exchange of information, experience, and scientific findings was the predominant objective of the networks (65.4 per cent or 34 networks), followed by advocacy (48.1 per cent or 25 networks), support to strategy development (38.5 per cent or 20 networks) and capacity building (26.9 per cent or 14 networks). Other objectives (19.2 per cent or 10 networks) included conducting situation analyses and needs assessments, promotion of collaboration/cooperation and/or identifying research needs.

TRNs and Knowledge Management

Knowledge management is the systematic dissemination, sharing and adaptation of information and experiences. Knowledge management systems are made so as to modify an organisation's effectiveness and efficiency. Most of the initial work on knowledge management was done in the for—profit sector, where efficiency is a major concern. Systems that help to get rid of such waste are attractive to the corporate sector. They are equally attractive to development organisations, specially for the transfer of internal knowledge and the dissemination of 'best practice'. For development agencies, programme managers and analysts working on HIV/AIDS, the most important issue is how to use optimally the growing collection of 'best practice' materials. TRNs facilitate this through the dissemination and adaptation of such best practices.

Knowledge management systems seem to work best when the people who generate the knowledge are also those who store it, explain it to others and coach them as they try to apply the knowledge. It has been well documented, however, that typical approaches to knowledge management actually widen the gap between knowing and doing.

How does Knowledge Management Widen the Gap between Knowing and Doing?

(a) Knowledge management efforts generally focus on technology and the transfer of codified information.

(b) Knowledge management tends to treat knowledge as a tangible item, as a stock or a quantity, and therefore separates the knowledge from its intended use.

(c) Formal systems cannot simply store or transfer knowledge that is not easily described or codified but is nonetheless important for doing the work called tacit knowledge.

(d) The people incharge of transferring and implementing knowledge management do not understand the actual work being documented very often.

(e) Knowledge management tends to emphasize on specific practices, while ignoring the importance of philosophy.

Source: Pfeffer J, Sutton R. *The knowing doing gap: how smart companies turn knowledge into action.* Harward Business School Press. Cambridge, MA. p. 22, 2000.

How the TRNs Serve as Effective Tools of Knowledge Management?

It is important to note that effective knowledge management involves sharing of skills in addition to sharing knowledge. How could TRNs serve as a mechanism for effective management of knowledge? First, we note that in the absence of proper information and knowledge, organisations (including governments) are less likely to make sound choices. Second, we turn to the social learning theory, according to which individuals learn from others whom they observe, and then imitate by following a similar (but not necessarily identical) behaviour. Such social modelling commonly occur through diffusion networks. By linking innovators with others who are tackling similar issues, TRNs can perform catalytic role in the diffusion of innovations for HIV/AIDS control - so-called diffusion networks (Rogers, 1999). Diffusion scholars have since long realized that an individual's decision about an innovation may not be an instantaneous act. Rogers (1995) presents a model of the innovation decision process described in the following paragraph. At the same time, similar ideas may arise in different places in response to related problems. TRNs brings together workers in different settings, enabling them to share ideas and tools for better performance in the fight against HIV/AIDS.

Formation and Managing of Networks

Formation, Funding and Management

Networks are formed as an answer to perceived needs. Forming a network usually requires immense motivation and effort from a small group of individuals or agencies. Sustaining a network can be equally challenging as the network's founders struggle to generate the funding, membership, activities and structure to ascertain that the network survives and grows. In light of these challenges, the International Council of AIDS Service Organisations (ICASO; www.icaso.org) identified eight key steps to building a network (ICASO, 1997), to which items 9 and 10 have been added in this document.

Model of the Innovation Design Process

Steps in building and sustaining a network

1. *Prepare a statement of purpose:* A statement of purpose is an accurate and agreed-upon statement of the reason for a network's existence, the values which underline the network and what the members want to accomplish.
2. *Define the goals and objectives:* A goal is a broad statement that explains the changes that members want to achieve through their actions. Objectives are specific, measurable statements of the desired changes that a network intends to achieve by a given time.

3. *Create an action plan:* An action plan is a set of steps that are developed to accomplish a specific objective. At the least an action plan should (a) identify the activities needed to achieve an objective, (b) identify resources, (c) delegate responsibilities to persons in the network, (d) set a timetable for actions and (e) implement, monitor and evaluate.
4. *Establish ground rules:* In the initial process of networking it is important to address the issue of how members of the networks are to interact with one another. ICASO has identified 13 examples of ground rules, of which the following are examples: (i) come to meetings ready to listen, ponder, debate and question, (ii) use your role in the network to build group strength, to enable decision making in which everyone can feel comfortable and (iii) keep informed about issues related to the work of the network, building your knowledge and understanding of all sides of the issue.
5. *Define a decision-making process:* Decisions can be made in various ways. Three typical forms of decision making in networks are command, consultative and consensus.
6. *Prepare a communication plan:* This directs the timely transmission and receipt of information. For formal communications within the network, members may select combinations of the following: meetings, newsletters, faxes, phone calls, e-mail or web-based discussion, informal communications among members are less structured, need to be inspired and never thwarted.
7. *Choose an organisation structure:* The key principle is that the structure should help the network to achieve its goals. In practice, this may need the creation of units, including committees or working groups, a coordination unit or secretariat, office staff and a decision-making body.
8. *Secure resources:* There are three major forms of resources needed for networking: money, people and contributions in-kind.
9. *Define responsibilities:* These include responsibilities for making and executing decisions, convening meetings, promoting communications and mobilizing resources.

10. *Develop monitoring and evaluation plan:* A monitoring and evoluation plan is needed to monitor progress toward set objectives and to enable corrective action where necessary.

Source: International Council of AIDS Service Organisations, HIV/AIDS Networking Guide. 1997, ICASO. Ottawa, pp. 9-17.

Challenges of Building Networks

Networks face mutlifarious challenges. They include: time constraints, limited funds, limited technical capacity at the local level, divergent views among funding institutions and technical barriers to the delivery of network services. How well these are resolved will affect the success of the network. Several networks have gone through the formative stages and achieved some of their objectives. They include the Africa-based Regional AIDS Training Network and the Asian Harm Reduction Network described as follows:

The Regional AIDS Training Network (RATN), Nairobi, Kenya

The Regional AIDS Training Network (RATN) is innovative and adds importance to country-level work. RATN includes 13 partner institutions and 9 affiliate institutions in Eastern and Southern Africa, working with WHO, EU as well as academic and research institutions in Belgium, Canada, Kenya and South Africa. As part of its benefits to African countries, RATN aids in curriculum development, identifies and supports regional training venues, and enables communications among institutions, trainers and trainees. By mid-1999, RATN had served 470 course participants from 17 African countries. Courses include AIDS counselling, management of STI, community care, communications, adult education, policy and planning, research methodology and laboratory management. RATN is gender-sensitive in the component of the course and in the mix of course participants. Former course participants now have a variety of responsibilities for community care and counselling in countries including Kenya, Malawi, Zambia and Zimbabwe.

Expected long-term effects includes: (a) strengthened potential of regional institutions to function as innovative centres for research and training in STI/HIV; (b) modified skills of STI/

AIDS workers in the region; (c) effective exchanges of strategies and information among countries in the region; and (d) modified care, and a reduction in the incidence of STI/HIV.

The Asian Harm Reduction Network (AHRN)

AHRN is a regional organisation that focuses on HIV and injecting drug use (IDU). This technical resource network has became an important means of promoting the harm reduction approach in Asia and strengthening HIV prevention among injecting drug users (IDUs).

Among other advantages to countries in the region, the network has proved to be an important resource and mechanism for developing and conducting national and multi-country training activities on HIV prevention and harm reduction. These activities are being carried out throughout Asia and have focused on policy makers, health workers, law enforcement officials, drug-treatment workers, government and non-government staff and others interested in harm reduction. Training is a useful approach through which AHRN has built capacity at the country level for responses to HIV and IDU.

Lessons Learnt

Some of the lessons in developing and managing AHRN are as follows:

(a) Having financed secretariat, staffed by a full-time coordinator (the executive director), was important to developing the network, servicing its membership and securing finance for subsequent years.
(b) Sustaining the network required long time, effort and patience from AHRN staff and management.
(c) Developing AHRN's activities, establishing its secretariat and securing finance required considerable professional skill.
(d) Having a broad funding base was crucial
(e) Cross-cultural adaptation of harm reduction strategies was crucial for their acceptance.
(f) Support from local organisations and individuals has been important to the network's recognition and success.

Information Technology and TRNs

E-mail discussion forums provide a chance for people to share ideas and information on various themes. Some of these forums are open, such as AF-AIDS and SEA-AIDS, which can be joined by any individual or organisation engaged in the area of HIV/AIDS or interested in the topic (to join, sign up through www.hivnet.ch/fdp/). These forums aim to encourage organisations and individuals to share experiences on HIV/AIDS, learn from the experiences of others or debate disputes of a topical nature. The e-groups set up by the UNAIDS Intercountry Team for Eastern and Southern Africa (ICT/ESA) aim to enable the flow of information and to help TRNs share best practices, research and issues emerging from countries as shown in the following para. 'E-groups' is a web-based application (www.egroups.com) provided free of charge to the user. There are essentially two services associated to the e-groups: a group e-mail address and distribution to the group; and a website with various functions that enable networking and information sharing among the group.

The services provided by the e-groups

(a) The Document Vault, where documents of interest can be uploaded and stored in the vault.
(b) Links to World Wide Web Pages of Interest.
(c) A chat section, which can be used for online meetings, etc.
(d) A database feature where the contact details of all the members can be stored.
(e) A calendar feature for arranging meetings.

TRNs and the Web: Focus on Eastern and Southern Africa

The UNAIDS Intercountry Team for Eastern and Southern Africa is enabling the use of information technology by technical resource networks. These networks are:

(a) The UNAIDS E-group: This serves as a means of sharing information among the ICT, the Country Programme Advisers, Junior Professional Officers, Theme Group Chairpersons and the Cosponsors of UNAIDS. This network is used to keep members informed on regional news and to share information on ICT activities at the national level that may benefit others.

(b) *The Religious E-group:* This was developed to support a core group of religious organisations to discuss community mobilization with regard to HIV/AIDS control. The e-group will be taken over by the Norwegian Church AID, which is also exploring the possibility of providing funds to members to cover their connectivity costs. On-going discussions address widening the core members by inviting other religious bodies to become involved in HIV/AIDS-related issues.

(c) *The Debt-for- AIDS E-group:* The e-group's aim is to share relevant information and perspectives with key stakeholders working on Debt-for-AIDS activities. Many countries with high HIV prevalence are also largely indebted to external institutions and governments. Debt service obligations diminish public funds that might otherwise be available for AIDS control programmes. Debt-for-AIDS seeks to mitigate poverty and support development by putting the AIDS control agenda in the key development instruments of these countries, including their Poverty Reduction Strategy Papers, debt relief agreements and Medium-Term Expenditure Frameworks. For countries qualifying for debt relief under the Heavily Indebted Poor Countries (HIPC) initiative, Debt-for-AIDS advocates that funds from debt relief be tied in part to AIDS control programmes, through short term actions and medium-term goals. Stakeholders include government representatives, civil society, U.N agencies and creditors. This e-group included 300 members as of mid-2000.

(d) *HIV/AIDS Media E-group:* This e-group is jointly controlled by UNAIDS and SAFAIDS and aims to provide journalists in the region with latest information on HIV/AIDS.

TRNs and the Electronic Network in the Asia-Pacific Region

The UNAIDS Asia-Pacific Intercountry Team (APICT) enables five electronic networks in support of technical resource networks. These networks are:

(a) *The UNAIDS APICT E-group (APICT-net):* A means of sharing informations among the UN family members in the Asia Pacific Region, specially Country Programme Advisers, Junior Professional Officers, UNAIDS Theme Group Chairpersons and the UNAIDS Cosponsors. This network is used to inform members on latest news (*AIDSFlash*) and events from the region, to share information on activities of APICT and the UNAIDS Cosponsors. *AIDSFlash* is a biweekly news service summarising the HIV/AIDS press from over 20 regional sources. It is sent to all networks supported by APICT and other interested networks/individuals.

(b) *The ASEAN Task Force on AIDS E-Group (ATFOAnet):* This e-group is jointly administered by UNAIDS and the AIDS Division of Thailand's Ministry of Public Health. The group provides members of the ASEAN Taskforce on AIDS with a platform to discuss issues, identify possible solutions and share experiences and information.

(c) *The Asian AIDS Information Network E-group (AAIN):* This e-group brings together organisations that are means of HIV/AIDS information to: share relevant information, experiences and resources between collaborating organisations; clearly specifies respective roles of individual resource centres, and to gives descriptions of services and materials available to clients in the region ; reduce duplication efforts in the provision of HIV information and materials; and enables the referral of clients to appropriate sources of good-quality information and materials. UNAIDS is presently negotiating with a resource centre based within the region to take over responsibility for the network.

(d) *The TB-HIV/AIDS E-group:* This e-group set up to facilitate the sharing of information, ideas, suggestions and concerns about the increased threat of TB-HIV/AIDS and to identify ways of applying social mobilization to expand the response to this 'deadly duet'.

(e) *SEA-AIDS:* Established in 1996, this network led electronic communication in the HIV/AIDS field in Southeast Asia. The e-mail discussion forum connects around 2400 people and organisations working in and with Asian Nations related to the epidemic. The forum facilitates people to discuss current HIV/AIDS issues, share experiences about what does and does not work in relation to the epidemic, as well as sharing news and forthcoming events.

Lessons Learnt

(a) Where there is a real felt need to exchange information (i.e. small group of technical experts working on a common area of concern), the e-group system is beneficial.

(b) In some cases the lack of communication may also be the consequence of the members themselves not being altogether sure how to use the technology.

(c) It is involves a lot of time to set up and maintains the database, links, documents, vault, etc. The e-group needs to be continuously updated to ensure that the member listing remains current. This is not necessarily the case in small technical e-groups. On the other hand, once this is in place it will be easier to manage the e-group and keep it going.

(d) Inspite of no cash costs apart from electricity and telephone access, a moderately skilled user is required to moderate an e-group.

(e) Being web-based (except for the e-mail function) could be problematic in those countries with inadequate telecommunications infrastructure. This is the case in many countries in Southern Africa and therefore finding the webpage on e-groups, with all the functions and options available, could be problematic.

(f) Some people just do not have the time to go through and answer all the e-mails. Moderated e-mail forums may need to convert messages into summaries, in order to present the informations concisely thereby reducing the time required to read them.

These lessons learnt and those identified by others are quite identical (Kumaranayake and Watts, 2000). The Internet, like any information communication technology, is not crucial to good information management. A TRN that has defined what information it requires and how information communication technology can be utilized to meet those needs will be far ahead of one which, is without thoughtful assessment of its objectives and needs, makes extensive use of computers, e-mail and the Internet.

A Programme for Action

TRNs are a means of speedening the spread of effective responses to HIV/AIDS. TRNs are complex systems and present challenges in the fields of management, financing, monitoring and evaluation. The UNAIDS Secretariat is working with its Cosponsors, bilateral agencies and regional institutions to reinforce on-going efforts to support networking, using the following mutually strengthening strategies.

Development of Resource Materials to Improve Networking

The UNAIDS Secretariat will provide interested parties with guidelines and reference materials to help them establish and manage TRNS. Material published include case studies of the Asian Harm Reduction Network, the Regional AIDS Training Network in Africa, the Latin American and Caribbean Strategic Planning Network and InfoDev, the electronic connectivity initiative in Southeast Asia. In order to provide networks with tools for effective management, UNAIDS plans to put together methodological experiences from these case studies into a single volume on the monitoring and evaluation of TRNs. As countries increase their programmes of action against HIV/AIDS, there is a growing needs for accelerating access to skilled persons to support programme development and implementation.

In response to this need, and with the approval of cosponsors and partner agencies, the UNAIDS Secretariat has developed a Directory of Technical and Managerial Resources, starting with those working on or in Africa. The data available on diskette and the UNAIDS website. The Directory has improved networking by making it easier for managers and analysts to identify institutions and persons with whom they need to establish professional contacts on a given subject.

Expanding the Knowledge Base

As political support for HIV/AIDS programmes increases, the UNAIDS Secretariat will explore ways to leverage such political support for increased funding. For example, the UNAIDS Secretariat is working with partner institutions, including the World Bank and USAID, to develop a toolkit (discussed in this book) on Debt-for-AIDS. As more finances become available for HIV/AIDS control, the concern in many countries will shift from that of a lack of finances to that of effective programming and efficient use of resources. In recognition this, UNAIDS is employed in equipping managers of National AIDS Control Programmes with tools and techniques for efficient allocation of resources. A new training module on priority-setting within HIV/AIDS programmes, focused on analysts and managers of national programmes and NGOs, was launched in the last quarter of 2000. These training materials will strengthen the work of AIDS strategic planning networks in Africa, Asia and Latin America.

Initiating and Supporting Networks

The UNAIDS Secretariat and Cosponsors will increase its support for existing networks and encourage the formation of new ones, stressing on their potential to affect the course of the epidemic. Such support could include technical inputs, start-up funds (usually modest and specially designed to garner larger resources from other sources), advocacy and information dissemination. A promising example is the Strategic Planning Network for Western and Central Africa, launched in Ouagadougou in August, 2000.

Facilitating Communication for Networking

In addition to the electronic discussion forums, UNAIDS is also developing on electronic workspace (eWorkspace) devoted to capacity-building and technical resource strengthening for HIV/AIDS programmes at the sub-regional and regional levels. The prototypes target is on Africa. This eWorkspace is a tool to develop, document and disseminate timely methods and examples in response to specific needs for technical support at the country and regional levels. It will employ expertise from UNAIDS Cosponsors, regional institutions, partner agencies and client countries. The Africa eWorkspace was launched in October, 2000.

References

International Council of AIDS Service Organisations. *HIV/AIDS Networking Guide,* 1997, ICASO. Ottawa, Canada.

Kumaranayake L, Watts C., Moderating discussions on the web: opportunities, challenges and lessons learned. *Health Policy and Planning;* 15(1): 116-118. 2000.

Powell M., *Information Management for Development Organisations.* 1999, Oxfam. Oxford, UK.

Pfeffer J, Sutton R. *The knowing-doing gap: how smart companies turn knowledge into action.* Harvard Business School Press. Cambridge, MA, United States. P 261. 2000.

Rogers E., *Diffusion of Innovations.* Second Edition, 1995. The Free Press, New York, United States.

Starkey P., Networking for development. International Forum for Rural Transport and Development, London, UK. ISBN 1 85339 430 0. 1997.

UNAIDS. Inventory of UNAIDS Networking Activities, Implications for Future Workplan. Unpublished report prepared for the UNAIDS Secretariat by Sara Kim. August, 1999.

Three

Social Marketing of Condoms

Social marketing projects and programmes exist in dozens of developing countries but, at the same time, there are still many more countries with the potential to adopt or expand similar activities. Since its inception in 1996, UNAIDS has promoted and supported social marketing, and especially the social marketing of condoms, as a key strategy in the fight against the spread of HIV/AIDS and STDs.

This study presents six applications of different social marketing techniques drawn from among on-going projects in developing countries in the field of reproductive health and prevention of HIV/AIDS and STDs. Individually they illustrate different, practical approaches to condom promotion through social marketing in response to particular challenges and needs. All applications describe activities from which important lessons may be learned. In addition, they demonstrate the versatility of social marketing and how the technique can be adapted to deal with differing situations and constraints.

The study is mainly useful for individuals and organisations, from both the public and private sectors, who are interested in learning more about social marketing, and how its concepts and techniques can be applied in response to the spread of HIV/AIDS and STDs, particularly in developing countries. It is aims at providing basic information, as an aid to training, programme planning and related activities.

Social Marketing - Meaning

"Social marketing" may be defined as the adaptation of commercial marketing and sales concepts and techniques to the attainment of social goals. It enables making health-related information, products and services easily available and affordable to low-income populations and those at risk while simultaneously promoting the adoption of healthier behaviour. In fact, it may be said that the ultimate goal of social marketing is to effect healthy and sustainable behaviour change.

One part of the social marketing equation is making quality products and services affordable and available. Encouraging their use represents the other. Market research and a strong communications component are essential for the success of a social marketing programme.

Social marketing has become very popular among governments and donors as an efficient and effective means of addressing serious health issues in developing countries. It has it origin in family planning but the concept is now applied across many fields in public life and health, in both developed and developing countries, including such areas as protection of the environment, campaigns against smoking and alcohol abuse, and the prevention and care of malaria, leprosy and tuberculosis. However, the use of social marketing for improving the sexual and reproductive health of women and men in developing countries has attracted particular attention. It is a means to complement and not replace (or even seek to replace), free access to health services and products. It therefore does not compete with the public health system and in fact support existing systems. By making low-cost products available outside the health system, social marketing programmes mitigates the pressure on existing services while allowing the health system to use limited resources more efficiently.

In the case of condoms, social marketing can be an alternative source of products and information for people who may be unable or unwilling to reach out locations where privacy is too often impaired. For instance, through social marketing condoms are widely available in places where people regularly go, as opposed to reproductive health clinics, which are much less frequented by men and young people. The possibility of anonymity in a commercial transaction then becomes attractive, particularly to women and sexually active young people. Government support, plays a key role in the success of social marketing programmes and these are often developed in close collaboration with host country government according to with national priorities and needs.

Many governments recognize the significant contributions of social marketing to improving the sexual and reproductive health of their low-income populations and extend important financial and political support to the activity. In many countries, for example, socially marketed products, generally condoms, are allowed tax exemptions or may be directly subsidized by local or national government in order to reduce costs and prices; other examples include the use of IEC (Information, Education and Communication) materials developed by social marketing in public schools and clinics, or the relaxation of restrictions on the use of mass media for educational communications on sexual and reproductive health issues. Until a few years back it was very rare to find a country where advertising of condoms was permitted in the mass media channels, something that has now become quite common.

Condom Social Marketing (CSM) Programmes

During mid-1980s, condom social marketing (CSM) emerged as an effective tool in the fight against, HIV/AIDS. Through social marketing programmes and projects in many countries affected by the epidemic condoms have become more easily available, affordable and acceptable to sexually active men, women and young people in general, as well as to those in high-risk groups. Although the programmes have generally focused on the product, accompanying communications and IEC activities have significantly contributed to raised awareness of the risks of infection and the means of prevention, reaching people, governments and institutions in all sectors of public and private life. Thus, Condom social marketing programmes have made condoms more accessible, affordable and acceptable in many of the world's poorest countries. In 1997 these distributed conetous to about 900 million males and females. By 1999, at least 71 different social marketing programmes for male and female condoms were active in 59 developing countries.

In the case of condoms social marketing has emerged as a

"normalizer" of the product, reducing the stigmas popularly attached to it. Until a few years back public access to condoms was difficult in many developing countries, as the product was often available only in pharmacies and health clinics and generally considered to be more appropriate for use by and with commercial sex workers. Now, thanks to years of constant social marketing activities, condoms are widely available in many countries from a variety of outlets, openly discussed in public and in the media, and are seen by many, including many of those at high risk of HIV infection, to be common household items. This "destigmatization" of condoms in many countries illustrates how social marketing can help populations to overcome social and cultural stigma in practising effective prevention of STDs and HIV/AIDS.

The Role of UNAIDS

The Joint United Nations Programme on HIV/AIDS (UNAIDS) is the leading proponent for global action on HIV/AIDS. UNAIDS leads, strengthens and supports an expanded response so as to prevent the transmission of HIV, providing care and support, reducing the vulnerability of individuals and communities, and minimising the impact of the epidemic. Since its establishment in 1996, UNAIDS has promoted and supported social marketing, and particularly the socialmarketing of condoms, as a key instrument in the fight against the spread of HIV and AIDS. UNAIDS plays a unique and important role in garnering support for social marketing programmes as a çosponsored programme.

At the national level, UNAIDS encourages governments and NGOs to support, develop and implement HIV/AIDS prevention social marketing initiatives within their countries. This may include recommending the inclusion of social marketing in national plans, the assignment of resources to social marketing programmes from multilateral and bilateral donors, and the facilitation of a positive legislative environment for social marketing. The exchange of servatrous between organisations and countries is also encouraged. In countries where social marketing programmes are being initiated, UNAIDS plans a big role as fundraiser and, more recently, as a potential provider of technical assistance in working with leading social marketing organisations, such as Population Services International (PSI) and suppliers of products, such as with The Female Health Company, sole manufacturer of female condoms. In addition, through its regional and country network of programme advisers, Theme Groups and co-sponsors, UNAIDS offers an excellent means of disseminating information, observations, best practices and lessons learned in social marketing.

UNAIDS stimulates social marketing in the following field

(a) Myanmar, the Russian Federation, Haiti, Cuba and Ghana
(b) Female condoms
(c) Application of social marketing to other HIV/AIDS-related products and services

UNAIDS promotes expanded interest in social marketing through:

(a) UNAIDS website
(b) Social marketing assessments in Bulgaria, Cuba, Guyana, Liberia, the former Yugoslav Republic of Macedonia, and Turkey
(c) Regional Marketing Training Exchange with projects in Albania and Romania
(d) Forum 2000 on Social Marketing (in development)

UNAIDS provides key resources such as best practice materials and case studies, including:

(a) "Social Marketing: An Effective Tool in the Global Response to HIV/AIDS"
(b) "Three Key Lessons Learned in Condom Social Marketing"
(c) "A Global Directory of Condom Social Marketing Projects and Programmes"

Approaches to Social Marketing

The existing commercial infrastructures in countries is generally used by social marketing programmes to develop and distribute specifically branded products such as condoms. This "traditional" approach, also called the "own brand model", is the most common amongst social marketing programmes in developing countries and is closely related to Population Services

International (PSI) and DKT International, organisations that pioneered international social marketing in the 1970s and 1980s. It applies standard commercial marketing and sales techniques for promotion and distribution through wholesale and retail outlets to the mass market. The social marketing organisation may receive unbranded goods from international or national donors, or may directly procure quality products from manufacturers, and develop its own brands and packaging for distribution. This includes the establishment of a professional in-country sales force and management structure, frequently involving a local partner organisation. The ability to function as effectively as possible in a wide variety of contexts is a key element in any social marketing programme. In most developing countries low-income populations form the great majority and among them there is a frequent need to target specific, often difficult to access, population groups with particular needs.

In addition to working through traditional sales networks involving wholesalers and existing retail outlets for consumer goods, social marketing programmes must frequently try to develop non-traditional outlets and informal distribution systems to meet the needs of special groups, and even communities, within the population. The possible use of alternative distribution systems is an essential aspect of social of social marketing. Nowadays in many developing countries, socially marketed condoms are found in both traditional retail outlets such as pharmacies and drugstores and non-traditional outlets such as bars, coffee shops, brothels, beauty parlours, workplaces, gas stations, and bus and truck terminals. Therefore, other ways of social marketing of products have been developed and are also common.

These approaches are not mutually exclusive although one or more may be applied exclusively by a programme or project, or also as parts of a project for strengthening and improvement of an existing "traditional" approach.

Types of Social Marketing

These models, or possible approaches to social marketing, include:

(i) Community-based systems of product promotion and distribution ("community-based distribution"/CBD).

Here non-professional sales agents are appointed from among particular groups within the general population. The individuals receive basic training in IEC (Information, Education and Communication) and sales and are usually rewarded financially from small margins on their sales. This approach is preferably chosen as a means of reaching geographical areas and socio-cultural groups that are difficult to access. Many programmes use the method to complement more traditional, retail outlet sales; some programmes, generally run by local NGOs, are based entirely on the system.

(ii) Community Based Social Marketing (CBSM) Network

An innovative and promising variant of the CBD method has recently been developed and steered over two years in Chennai, India, by International Family Health (IFH) and its local partner NGO, the Indian Institute of Community Health (IICH). In this approach ("community-based social marketing"/CBSM) sales agents are appointed from among the general public as well as from within specific groups. In addition to taking advantage of basic training in reproductive health and from commissions on their sales, the agents also benefit financially from recruiting others to act as educational and sales agents. CBSM originated from commercial "network" and "multi-level" marketing techniques successfully applied in developed countries, and has shown possibilities of success in rapidly attaining community penetration and involvement in reproductive health issues and HIV prevention.

(iii) Supporting the Manufacturer through Grants

The "manufacturer's model" where support is provided for the promotion and distribution of brands produced and owned by a manufacturer (foreign or local) or local manufacturer's agent, frequently an importer of the product. The support is in the form of grants directly to the manufacturers and/or their distribution agents so as to reduce their commercial marketing costs and therefore allow greater investment in key activities, such as promotion and advertising.

(iv) Targeted Services Delivery Approach

The "targeted service delivery" approach includes planning suitable social marketing activities, through which the project tries to reach and distribute products to specific target groups, usually high-risk or other priority groups of the general public. Who are often inadequately served by other service delivery mechanisms, including standard social marketing activities. Their identification are made from market segmentation studies carried out once the basic distribution structure to the mass market is established. Thus, targeted service delivery is often a component of programmes mainly structured around the "traditional" or wider commercial approach. However, many local organisations, usually NGOs, adopt this approach either from need (due to restricted resources) or from particular interest.

There are many ways of applying social marketing concepts, models and techniques at the national, local or community levels. Flexibility in planning and implementation are important in successfully meeting the needs for information and products such as condoms in the fight against the spread of HIV and AIDS. Planning and putting into effect the social marketing programmes is by no means restricted to large, well-funded international organisations. Local initiatives in social marketing by organisations within the national "private sector", including NGOs, are there many countries. These differ widely in size and purpose from small, localized projects restricted, to training and employing ex-commercial sex workers in a particular location as sales and IEC agents only for condoms, to large, full-scale reproductive health programmes active at the national level.

The fact that well-managed and adequately supported social marketing projects are among the most cost-effective of health interventions is of particular interest to local initiatives. The projects can get back a large proportion of costs and revenues from sales which can be invested in other activities, such as capacity-building or strengthening the programme itself if the organisation works wholly in social marketing (the Social Marketing Company of Bangladesh, for example). If the organisation has other activities, as does PROFAMILIA in Colombia then these revenues can also be used to subsidize these activities within a policy of cross-subsidization. The following two case studies of social marketing applied to the prevention of HIV/AIDS and STDs in different countries and contexts elucidate the various approaches described above. The cases described are examples of the uses of these models to social marketing that have been adopted in some countries by different organisations; all the cases focus on methods of condom distribution and promotion that were designed and implemented in response to varied circumstances.

CASE STUDY-1

Haiti—Relevant Facts

Haiti has a total land area, consisting of 27600 square kilometres of mountainous terrain and a total estimated population of 8.1 million of whom almost 70 per cent live in rural areas.

It is the poorest of the Latin American and Caribbean countries having a GNP per capita of US$ 250 in 1995 estimated by the World Bank. The vast majority of the population live on subsistence incomes, mainly from agriculture. Haiti ranks 156 on UNDP's Human Development Index and life expectancy at birth is 54 years, much lower than the regional average of 70 years.

The occurrence of HIV infection amongst Haitians aged 15-49 years is estimated at 5.17 per cent by the end of 1999, which is amongst the highest in the region, with an estimated 2,10,000 people living with HIV/AIDS and 23,000 deaths due to AIDS in 1999. Already by the late 1980s HIV prevalence among sex workers tested in major urban areas ranged from 42 per cent to 53 per cent. The prevalence of STD is very high, and a 1992 study of male STD clinic patients found that 25 per cent of patients tested were HIV-positive.

Application of Community-based Distribution (CBD) Approach in Haiti and Mozambique

The use of sales agents drawn from the community and trained in IEC and condom promotion and sales is crucial to the performance of the condom social marketing programmes in several countries, Haiti and Mozambique being among them. However, the main reasons for adopting this strategy, either on its own or complementing other forms of condom distribution, may differ as also the forms it takes may differ. The examples of Haiti and Mozambique not only illustrate the potential effectiveness of CBD systems in condom social marketing, but also suggests different reasons for the choices and different ways of working by CSM programmes. In both countries the social marketing programmes must deal with the problems involved in making condoms easily accessible and distributed to largely rural populations and communities.

In Haiti the mountainous terrain, interspersed with valleys inhabited by semi-isolated communities and served by a precarious transportation system, was a key factor in the decision to recruit sales agents from the communities through existing local NGOs. The agents work to strengthen a system consisting of traditional commercial distribution based on an existing commercial network for other consumer goods. Substantial amounts of condom sales are made through the community-based distributors (CBDs), though traditional distribution accounts for most of the volume.

In Mozambique, on the other hand the existence of large communities, isolated by the geographical terrain, was not as problematic as the fact that many years of civil war had devastated the national infrastructure for transportation and communications as well as the economy and a commercial sector which was just making a beginning. Standard distribution of products was thus extremely difficult, even in urban areas, and there was no commercial distribution "up-country". It was decided to lay stress initially on establishing a distribution system based on a network of locally recruited and trained sales and motivation teams. One team was initiated per province; the role of the motivation agent was focused on creating demand for condoms (particularly amongst high-risk groups through interpersonal communications activities), whereas the equally important role of the sales agent was to meet the demand by supplying the retailer. This was necessary due to the fact that condoms in Mozambique were still comparatively new and unknown product. A more formal, traditional means of distribution through a wholesaler-retailer chain could emerge over time. In 1999, 49 per cent of sales were to community agents, 34 per cent to commercial distributors and 16 per cent to workplaces and NGOs. The proportion of sales to community agents in the year 2000 is expected to be 45 per cent and further decrease is expected as the commercial sector grows.

Social Marketing for AIDS Prevention: Haiti

Population Services International (PSI) has been conducting social marketing for reproductive health and reduction in high-risk sexual behaviour in Haiti since 1989, working on providing accessible and affordable condoms to the low-income segments of the population for HIV/STD prevention. By the end of 1996, two branded condoms (one male, one female) were successfully launched on to the market and other contraceptive products (pills and injectables) were added to the range of products. As geographical, economic and political conditions in Haiti make it very difficult to implement a social marketing programme of regular product distribution through the commercial wholesaler-to-retailer structure adopted in most countries. In Haiti the majority of the population lives in rural areas that are not easily approachable due to the mountainous terrain and a precarious infrastructure of roads and transportation. The vast majority of the population has little or no regular income Political instability and unrest is a constant aspect of daily life. Under these circumstances it was decided in 1990 to start a supplementary programme for creating a system based on the sale of products, mainly male condoms, together with related IEC activities. This was carried out through trained individuals, locally recruited from the communities and population groups targeted by the overall programme, i.e. a system of community-based distributors, and motivated by a substantial financial incentive usually with a commission on sales.

Advantages of CBD and Social Marketing

(a) *Credibility:* as relatives, friends and neighbours are more welcome than salespeople from outside;
(b) *Availability:* as CBDs are accessible at any time of the day or night;
(c) *Privacy and discretion:* where condoms are available on a personal basis;
(d) *Effective counselling:* dealing with individual needs and, ensuring correct and consistent use.

For achieving this, PSI/Haiti formed a partnership with nine local NGOs, with wide access to rural communities, and created and registered its own NGO. PSI trained 175 members of the NGOs in topics like STDs and HIV/AIDS prevention, social marketing goals and strategies, interpersonal communication and direct sales techniques, condom use demonstrations and basic money management. After the training they were qualified to work as wholesale distributors selling to retail outlets and as retail sales agents to consumers.

After training, each CBD was provided with a free stock of condoms, up to 10 retail dispensers each containing 144 condoms, in order to begin selling. With the resulting income, repurchase more supplies after retaining an agreed margin. Initially it was thought that some CBDs might prefer to sell their condoms to higher-income groups rather than their targeted populations and, also, that the IEC binding of the CBD role might be neglected in favour of sales. While monitoring the activities of many CBDs PSI/Haiti discovered that, some were in fact selling condoms to more affluent people, but they were not neglecting their target groups who reported that condoms were available whenever needed. The dramatic increase in sales recorded showed that individuals were being convinced to purchase and use condoms, indicating that the IEC function was being carried out.

The project was very successful. In all, more than 3000 points of sale for male condoms were established throughout Haiti, ensuring distribution to hundreds of thousands of customers and including other than traditional markets and commercial sales outlets, bars, hotels and even beauty salons in both urban and remote rural areas. The first four years showed a monthly sales of male condoms increased from 3000 to over 400000 pieces and continues to increase. It least 33 per cent of total sales through all channels employed in Haiti were due to CBDs, and a large share of regular sales outlets were opened by these individuals.

Moreover, by the end of 1996, between 70 and 95 per cent of sexually active adults, including 85 per cent of adolescent males, 70 per cent of adolescent females and 95 per cent of commercial sex workers, knew about "Pante" and recognized that condoms protect against AIDS. In 1998 nearly one in five women reported having used condoms specifically for STD/HIV protection. At the same time, however, survey results show that both awareness and use are still lower than could be expected in rural areas and that efforts must be maintained or even increased.

Constraints Encountered by CBDs

According to reports from PSI/Haiti, the main constraints and obstacles encountered included:

(a) Rapport between NGOs and social marketing in promoting HIV prevention is not automatic.

(b) It was simpler for NGO sales people to sell to more affluent customers in the cities than to the remote rural targets, and to confine their activities to selling instead of meeting their educational obligations.

Under the uncertain environment of military coup in 1991 highly motivated CBDs provided stability to the project, by attempting to continue their work despite the problems and dangers, and continuing to open up new sales outlets and share information on AIDS and its prevention.

Lessons Learnt

CBDs can make very significant contributions to both condom availability and accessibility, although individual performance may differ.

CBDs help in opening new sales regions and outlets that will be regularly serviced later by the professional sales force.

The direct costs to the organisation of adding CBDs to its sales force, is small compared to the benefits. However, more supervision and management time is required, particularly in the first months of operations. Professional Salespersons entail higher costs.

Even small margins on sales can be an incentive to CBDs. The income generated should be personal and not remitted to an organisation to which the CBD might belong.

NGOs and community-based organisations (CBOs) should not include this activity as a source of income. The NGOs are much better equipped to reach non-traditional outlets than commercial distributors.

Condom brand promotion is more successful when accompanied by mass media IEC as well as interpersonal, community-based condom promotion campaigns.

Maximum support from government and international agencies was also required. PSI need to function through NGOs as well as through commercial distributiors to function effectively in Haiti.

Condom Social Marketing (CSM) Haiti Project Information

(i) Project Duration

Initially the project was from 1991 to 1996, but due to continued funding to continued through 1999.

(ii) Implementing Agencies

(a) At the national level: programme de Sante et Information (PSI/Haiti), with the direct involvement of four national NGOs, and in partnership with the Ministry of Public Health and Population.

(b) At international level: Population Services International (PSI) and USAID (AIDSCAP).

(iii) Funding Agencies

USAID; alongwith the Government of the Netherlands, PSI Partnership Fund, world Bank, UNFPA, UNAIDS, the Bergstrom Foundation and the Summit Foundation.

(iv) Project Objectives

It aimed at reducing high-risk sexual behaviour and thus the transmission of HIV/AIDS. The main objectives were to:

(a) Target low income populations by making affordable condoms;

(b) Create awareness based consumer demand, consistent condom use;

(c) Reduce the occurrence of other STDs which significantly facilitate the transmission of (e.g. gonorrhoea, syphilis, and chlamydial infection) HIV/AIDS.

(v) Target Areas

The whole country, specially the rural areas where 70 per cent of the population live, and where access to condoms and other products is very limited. More than 3000 points of sale, were created through CBDs, and through them to non-traditional retail outlets like night clubs, bars and beauty salons.

(vi) Target Audience

General and high-risk populations, especially young people (age group 15 to 24 years), including female commercial sex workers, migrants and transport workers.

(vii) Condom Marketing

The PSI-branded male condom, "Kapot Pante" ("Panther"), is available nationwide at a low price of US$0.07 for a packet of three which is an affordable price for a population with an estimated per capita annual income of US$ 400. This price is roughly 10 times lower than the commercial brands. Intensive mass advertising depicted the "Pante" as denoting strength and masculinity. National media were heavily involved in promoting condoms for the prevention of AIDS and in addition, education of the client was an integral part of the work of each CBD. Trends show that the Carnival period (January to April) is the highest risk period for sexual transmission of disease. PSI/Haiti ended the millennium with a highly successful campaign to make "Carnival 2000" the safest since HIV and AIDS came to Haiti.

For additional information on this programme:

PSI/Haiti
Rue Theodule #1
Burdon Port-au-Prince
Haiti

Mozambique — Relevant Facts

Mozambique has a land area of 801,600 square kilometres with a total estimated population of 19.3 million of whom 66 per cent live in rural areas; 56 per cent of the population is below the age of 20. The capital, Maputo, has an estimated population of 2.2 million which consists of varied groups with several major languages but Portuguese is widely spoken and is the official language; male/female literacy rates are estimated at 58/23 per cent. The principal religions are indigenous beliefs (60 per cent) and Christianity (30 per cent). Being one of the poorest countries in the world with a GNP per capita in 1995 estimated to be US$ 80 the country ranks 166 on UNDP's Human Development Index. Half of the national income is from agriculture. Life expectancy at birth is estimated at 47 years, below the average for Africa of 51 years.

The occurrence of HIV infection amongst adults in Mozambique was estimated at 13.2 per cent by the end of 1999 which is among the highest in Africa, with 12,00,000 people living with HIV/AIDS and 98,000 deaths due to AIDS in 1999. By 1996 HIV prevalence among antenatal women tested in different locations across the country was found to be between 18 per cent and 23 per cent; in addition, the prevalence of STD is very high and by 1995, studies of male STD clinic patients found that between 23 per cent and 40 per cent of those tested were HIV-positive.

"Communications and Condom Marketing for AIDS Prevention: the promotion of safer sex among high-risk individuals in Mozambique"

With the end of its civil war in 1992, HIV transmission rates rose dramatically in Mozambique with the return of refugees from neighbouring countries where HIV prevalence had been higher than in Mozambique. The government had a project of free distribution of condoms which was severely affected by the years of civil war and prospects for improvement were thin. In 1994 the government's National AIDS Control Programme (NACP) invited PSI International to design and launch an AIDS prevention social marketing programme to promote safer sexual behaviour and the use of condoms. The overall aim of PSI was to improve the health of sexually active men and women and their children by reducing transmission of HIV/AIDS and other STDs.

Objectives of the Project

The project which was launched in early 1995 had two specific objectives:

(a) Increase the use of condoms, specially among persons vulnerable to HIV transmission, through the introduction, promotion and sale of a condom particularly developed for social marketing in Mozambique ("JeitO", the condom brand name).

(b) Increase the demand for condoms through the launch of

an integrated behaviour change communications system which would promote safe sex, while targeting high-risk groups such as commercial sex workers, long-distance truck drivers, STD clinic attendees, night club patrons, military and police, people with varied sex partners, youth (in and out of school) and women.

Criteria For Choosing Districts in Priority for the Project

Beginning in 1995 and working alongwith the National AIDS Control Programme, out of the total of 140 districts in Mozambique, 71 priority districts for AIDS prevention were then identified based on the following criteria:

(a) High incidence of STDs;
(b) Common borders with high HIV prevalence countries;
(c) High volume of trucking;
(d) High urban population density; and
(e) High incidence of returning refugees and migrant labourers.

There were 65 Community Agents (CAs) recruited and trained from these districts. They were trained in interpersonal communications (for example, each CA conducts 15 small group discussions every month with project target groups) and in sales techniques for "JeitO" condoms, focusing on ensuring access to these by high-risk groups through non-traditional outlets. The CAs are given a monthly stipend for their work in communications and, additionally, a margin from their sales of condoms. The CAs are monitored by the PSI Provincial Sales/Motivation agent. They are also regularly evaluated and provided with refresher training when necessary. New CAs are appointed and trained as vacancies are filled whilst maintaining the total of 65.

Factors Necessary For Behaviour Change

The CAs have a crucial role in the overall project strategy. They promote behaviour change, i.e. correct and consistent use of condoms, reduction in the number of sexual partners, treatment of STDs and, particularly for young people, sexual abstinence until marriage. The project evolved a framework based on six factors deemed necessary for behaviour change to occur: (i) Personal understanding of being at risk; (ii) Education on condoms; (iii) Existence of a conducive, supportive environment; (iv) Ready access to condoms; (v) Self-efficacy, or having the resolve and skills to take preventive action; and (vi) Appropriate condom brand positioning: the "JeitO" brand concept.

The project developed activities developed to affect each of the factors based on information obtained from the different target groups. The activities are designed around a mutually strengthening media mix, emphasizing interpersonal communications (drama, theatre and small group discussions) together with mass media (radio and TV spots, music videos and cassettes) and promotional materials. The project has eight theatre groups trained to direct five different targeted plays in every province of Mozambique, and on any given day, five plays are expected to be performed somewhere in the country. The results have been encouraging, with an estimate of 50 000 peer education AIDS/STD sessions having been held. They reached about 1 million members of the target population. In addition, 150 traditional healers and some traditional birth attendants have been trained in promoting the use of condoms among their clients. A KAP survey conducted in 1997 in urban and periurban areas revealed that 87 per cent of respondents were aware that condoms exist, 31 per cent had used condoms at least once and 78 per cent cited condoms as a means of preventing HIV infection (as against 38 per cent in a similar survey in Malawi).

More than 3000 condom sales outlets have been opened nationwide. The include non-traditional outlets for condoms in Mozambique such as bars and clubs, kiosks and tobacconists, gas stations, market stalls, NGOs, supermarkets, street vendors, "traditional healer" outlets and within workplaces. Demand for and sales of socially marketed condoms increased dramatically, although sales were affected by a shortage of subsidized product during 1998.

Constraints Encountered by Communication and Condom Marketing for AIDS Prevention

According to reports from PSI/Mozambique, the main constraints and obstacles encountered included:

(a) As the "JeitO" package of four condoms is sold to consumers for the equivalent of US$ 0.08 and condoms are still donor-supported; therefore in 1998 there was a shortage of subsidized condoms due to donor shortfall.

(b) PSI in Mozambique is seen as an international organisation in spite of the fact that the management of the project is 98 per cent Mozambican.

Lessons Learnt

Government can be an active partner in social marketing and even incorporate it in its own programmes. This is being done with the NACP in Mozambique where the condom social marketing project is a component of the national HIV prevention strategy. The government acknowledge the need for coordinating free condom distribution through the national health system with the social marketing project, bringing condoms to the entire population irrespective of the individual client's purchasing power. This is an objective of the current NACP strategic plan.

The principal criteria for the success of the project has been the emphasis given to involving the community in sales and promotion, right down to individual input through peer education and direct promotion at points of sale.

The success of the project has been largely due to its intensive promotional activities - not only through the media and theatre performances, but also by the individual community-based promotion by sales outlets, CAs, peer educators and traditional practitioners.

NACP Project (Mozambique) Project Information

(i) Project Duration

Pilot project in 4 provinces, 2 years from 1995 to 1996. Phase I, extended to national scale, 3 years 1997 to 1999. Phase II, planned for a further 3 years.

(ii) Implementing Agencies

(a) at national level National AIDS Control Programme, Ministry of Health, PSI/Mozambique, national media.
(b) at international level: PSI/Washington, USAID.

(iii) Funding Agencies

For the pilot study and Phases I and II, USAID and the Government of the Netherlands, with the addition of UK/DFID from 2000.

(iv) Target Areas

Pilot project in 4 provinces (Maputo, Sofala, Manica and Tete). Phase I, extension to national level. By December 1996, the project was functional in all 10 provinces, and by December 1998, the national structure was fully consolidated.

For additional information on this programme:
PSI/Mozambique,
Av. Patrice Lumumba 204,
C.P. 4059,
Maputo, Mozambique

Four

Dimensions of Expanded Response to HIV/AIDS

In continuation with the ongoing fight against AIDS/HIV there is sufficient evidence to prove that well designed programmes can mitigate the incidence of HIV/AIDS. Therefore new initiatives as being taken apart from strengthening of the already existing ones thus aiming towards a gradual decline in the incidence of HIV. It has been more than a decade and a half since the beginning of the HIV/AIDS epidemic and over a decade after the foundation of the Global AIDS Strategy[1] still a dual gap continues to grow unabatedly between the quick spread of the HIV epidemic and the small number of prevention efforts; and between the rising needs for care, support, and impact-alleviation, and the insufficient response to these needs[2]. Towards the end of 1997, over 30 million people had HIV/AIDS, including 12.1 million women, 17.4 million men and 1.1 million children. In 1997 itself 5.2 million adult women and men and about 600,000 children newly acquired HIV infection. The death due to AIDS-related illnesses in 1997 alone was 20 per cent of the total AIDS-related deaths since the beginning of the epidemic. Globally, these infections are spread almost equally among women and men. The developing world accounted for most of all new HIV infections in 1997. As the HIV pandemic pursues its course relentlessly, it has become fragmented and now consists of multiple, concurrent epidemics. Its effect is particularly severe on the developing world and on marginalized populations in industrialized countries.

The rate at which the HIV infections are growing and the pace at which HIV infection grows into AIDS have begun to decline in certain populations in some parts of the world. This is simultaneous to the adopting of safer behaviour alongwith this prevention and care services are expanding, and particularly in richer countries due to the availability of some retroviral therapies. By now enough knowledge and experience has been gained from prevention and care efforts advocating that the rate of transmission of HIV can be reduced and the onset of AIDS-related problems can be delayed significantly if well designed and sustainable programmes are undertaken. The response to the epidemic has not fully benefited from this accumulated knowledge. Very few partnerships exist among those participating in this response. Joint 'scaled-up' action is lacking. And the involvement of civil society in the design and implementation of HIV/AIDS programmes is restricted. Ongoing initiatives tend to target on responding to urgent needs for prevention, but for most of the affected populations, these responses are insufficient. Even more importantly they have not focused sufficiently on strategies for providing HIV/AIDS care and social support and for mitigating the impact; they have also declined from addressing the root causes of the epidemic in societies and communities. HIV and AIDS continue to affect certain individuals and communities more than others as a result of inadequate services and societal constraints. It has been accepted by now that HIV and AIDS will soon be part of our lives, even if sometime in the future we may have an inexpensive and highly effective vaccine and are able to ensure coverage, and despite antiretroviral therapies showing some effect in parts of the world. To prevent the HIV/AIDS epidemic and reduce its impact we need to expand the response considerably. This expansion has two elements. Firstly, the enchancement and improvement in the quality, scope and coverage of continuing prevention, care, support and impact-alleviation efforts focusing on individuals and populations seen to be at particular risk should happen at the same time. Secondly, these must be combined with actions directed towards societal factors that lower people's vulnerability to HIV/AIDS.

Risk and Risk Alleviation

With respect to HIV, risk is defined as the probability that a person may acquire HIV infection. Certain behaviours create, enhance and continue such risk, these include unprotected sex with a partner whose HIV status is unknown, multiple unprotected sexual partnerships, lack of following of infection-control guidelines in the health-care setting, repeated blood transfusion, especially of untested blood, and injecting drug use with shared needles and syringes. Prevention, care, support and impact-alleviation activities, guided by research findings, are inseparable elements of a meaningful response to HIV/AIDS. The success of prevention depends partly on reinforcing the capacities of communities, and of the health, economic, educational, social welfare, political and other systems to meet the needs of those who live with HIV and AIDS and those affected by HIV/AIDS. Risk arises from individuals engaging in risk-taking behaviour due to a number of reasons. They may, for instance, lack knowledge about HIV, they may be unable to carry on safer sex, they may perceive that HIV/AIDS affects a different social strata than their own, or they may not have access to condoms. A strong premise influencing programme planning so far has been that risk can be mitigated to a large extent if knowledge, attitudes and skills of individuals are influenced to allow adoption of safer behaviour.

A man having unprotected sex with multiple partners is an example of conscious risk-taking behaviour. The spouse/partner of this man may herself be faithful to him not knowing of his multiple partnerships or unable to ask him to take appropriate measures to protect against HIV infection. Both partner thus indulge in risk-taking behaviour when they have unprotected sex with each other. The initial response to HIV was targeted at reduction in risk-taking behaviour through aiming at individuals and groups. Examples of such targeted response include the provision of information and education, the promotion of condoms; the containment and early treatment of sexually transmitted diseases, needle and syringe exchange among drug-injecting population; and programmes to increase women's and young people's drive to demand their own protection when the balance of power between them and their sexual partners is not in their favour. These strategies have also aimed at increasing the safety of medical practices, including blood transfusion, in the health-care setting.

Traditional Ways of Risk Reduction

The control of communicable diseases has traditionally depended on:

(a) influencing individual decisions to adopt protective behaviours and practices;
(b) biomedical or physical interventions to mitigate the risk of the transmission of infectious agents; and,
(c) in some cases, legal action or use of force.

This is how smallpox was eradicated, several vaccine-preventable diseases were brought under control and food-borne diseases were contained. With almost two decades into the HIV epidemic, rational notions of risk have influenced programme planners. The complexities of risk-taking behaviour, however, may be overlooked by assuming that behaviour is always rational. Personal intimacy and interpersonal relations have a major effect on behaviour. An injecting drug user may 'choose' to share needles as it is an expression of cooperation with the drug-using support system; sharing may increase group identity and support as well as ensure shelter and the next 'fix'. A sex worker who protects herself with clients may have unprotected sex with her steady partner to show love and confidence in him.

This, the above measures have resulted in a decline in the HIV/AIDS epidemic in some populations, and that they need to be strengthened. However, the effect of such measures will differ depending on the quality of messages, the scope and diversity of the method used, the ability to target audiences, the existence and quality of accessible services, and the societal focus within which such efforts take place. From a public health point of view societal factors are considered when examining and predicting the risks that expose an individual to a particular disease. Public health interventions, however, have greatly targeted the individual, overlooking societal issues that may be at the root of ill health.

The response to HIV/AIDS, however, has broadened over the recent years to target not only on individual risk-taking behaviour, but also on the immediate environmental and societal factors that affect such behaviour, and the influence exerted by families and communities on individual behaviour. In many societies, important decisions, like those related to child-bearing, often involve the family, rather than only the individual or the couple, with the influence of elders being particularly strong. More importantly, there is a growing acceptance of the key role that power relationships and social inequities play in influencing risk. Over and above the concept of risk and risk-taking behaviour is thus the broader sphere of vulnerability and vulnerability reduction. Individual risk is seen, through this point of view, as influenced by societal factors that increase and continue the vulnerability of certain individuals and sections of society more than others. This acceptance merits a response to HIV/AIDS that goes beyond the immediate risk-taking act and the immediate environmental factors affecting it, to mitigating underlying factors that create an overall climate in which such risk-taking behaviours are encouraged, maintained and prove difficult to change[3]. In widening the response, the individual, familial and community aspects need to be looked into more comprehensively and in a complementary fashion. With respect to the reference of community a community is defined here as an association of people sharing a common interest or objective, rather than a geographical community alone. People, thus, belong to a wide of communities, for instance neighbourhood, sports club, local women's club, or religious groups. Gate-keepers and opinion leaders, e.g. political or religious leaders, influence the information coming into the community and community decisions.

Vulnerability and its Reduction

From a health point of view, vulnerability results from societal factors that affect adversely one's potential to exercise control over one's own health. A person who may not be highly sensitive to HIV today may become so tomorrow due to various reasons like the loss of employment causing stress, forced displacement and resultant disintegration of social support systems. The effect may not be the same for all. For example, for a member of a larger, extended family in rural India, the loss of employment may not necessarily lead to the above, consequences to the same degree as a person in more industrialized and urban environment,. Thus, the concept of vulnerability includes personal and external factors, a temporal dimension, and a complex interaction between these factors that may vary across cultures and within societies. With respect to HIV/AIDS, vulnerability is influenced by the interaction of a range of factors including (a) personal factors; (b) factors connected to the quality and coverage of services and programmes targeted at prevention, care, social support and impact-alleviation; and (c) societal factors. In combination, these factors may create or increase individual vulnerability, and as a result, collective vulnerability to HIV/AIDS; others may have a positive effect on reducing vulnerability.

Factors Affecting Vulnerability

Analysing vulnerability to HIV/AIDS includes not only identifying these factors, but also understanding how these factors interact with each other, and how they vary across contexts and cultures. *Personal factors* include, for instance: sexual history (number of partners, number of unprotected sexual acts, and nature of sexual act), access to knowledge and skills required to protect oneself and others and, in context of care and social support, awareness about treatment and social support programmes as well as skills to access and benefit from them. Membership of specific social networks may also affect this vulnerability. Factors *related to service and programmes* that influence vulnerability consist of for instance, the cultural inadequacy of HIV/AIDS programmes, the non-availability of such services due to distance, cost and other factors, and the lack of capacity of health systems to react to a growing demand for care and support for people with HIV/AIDS and those affected. Examples of *societal factors influencing vulnerability* include cultural norms, laws or social practices and beliefs that act as hindrances to essential prevention messages-on the promotion of condoms, the importance of safer sex, etc. such societal factors result in the inclusion, neglect or social exclusion of people on purpose depending on their private lifestyle, behaviours or choices, and more importantly due to socio-cultural characteristics.

Almost all over the epidemic has disproportionately affected individuals and communities who are left out or discriminated against for reasons of sex, age, ethnicity, race, sexuality, economic status, and cultural, religious or political affiliation. To mitigate the vulnerability of such individuals and communities of HIV/AIDS, it is specially necessary that the response be widened beyond risk-reduction strategies.

Stigmatization for reasons of sexuality, sexual behaviour, substance use or the mere fact of being HIV positive has increased the HIV epidemic since its emergence. Public fear of HIV/AIDS further strengthens stigmatization towards people who, for social, racial, behavioural or any other reasons, are associated with higher risk of acquiring HIV infection. This stigmatization can limit the reach to appropriate HIV prevention, care and support for people who may be most in need.

Young people of both sexes compose most of the current HIV infections in the world today. Their experience indicates how the combination of personal, service-related and societal factors discussed earlier can influence vulnerability. During the passage from childhood to adulthood, some young people may experience feelings of 'invulnerability' as well as a desire to experiment. They may also not be having knowledge on subjects such as sex and drugs. As a result they may knowingly or unknowingly take risks that expose them to infection. From a *service perspective,* young people may use paediatric services or adult health clinics, none of which are fully equipped to meet their specific needs, sensitive to young women's and men's development, and ensure confidentiality and quality health care. From a *societal perspective,* young people are observed to have limited rights and are expected to adhere to norms established for them until they day when (sometimes four or five years after the average age of sexual onset) they can claim full legal freedom. Their right to confidentiality is often violated, their access to information is limited and their sexuality is repressed.

Off late, some progress has been made in understanding the multiple reasons and manifestations of *gender inequality,* with greater acceptance of specific actions that can be undertaken. In the absence of policies and programmes that help in bridging the gender gap, many HIV/AIDS-related efforts may prove to be ineffectual and short-lived. Equal access to education, fair income distribution, sharing of ownership, equal employment opportunities and wages, equality before the law and in the area of customary practices are some of the specific actions that can reduce the gender power gap effectively. Many of these changes need efforts at the legal and policy level, as well as challenging predominant cultural norms[4].

Poverty is another factor which increases vulnerability to HIV. The growing rates of HIV/AIDS in economically deprived communities of the industrialized world and in developing countries highlight the role played by poverty in fuelling the epidemic. Since long there has been worldwide recognition of the negative effect of poverty on health and of the need to undertake strong action towards poverty reduction and development.

Internal economic disparity is as crucial as the overall level of wealth in reference to vulnerability. Violations of rights, physical and mental abuse, sexual exploitation, and withdrawal of rights further aggravates the gap between those who benefit from economic growth and those who suffer its ill effects. All these factors fuel the epidemic.

Development policies and programmes also could have positive and negative effects on the spread and impact of HIV/AIDS. Thus, it is crucial during the social planning process to think carefully on these potential after effects. This would be the position of an economic development initiative that would increase disproportionately the economic gap between its immediate beneficiaries and others. The latter being more vulnerable to HIV/AIDS owing to increasing marginalization on economic grounds and the need for support from alternative means of livelihood which may expose them to the risk of HIV/AIDS.

Designing interventions and policies that address vulnerability is complicated due to the interaction between factors such as gender and poverty which may alleviate only some aspects of vulnerability in some contexts, but it may enhance vulnerability in other contexts. For instance while data indicate that, in most cultures, poverty worsens the conditions in which HIV is transmitted, there is proof to suggest that the pattern is not uniform. There are emerging epidemics among the better-off sections of society partly due to the economic power to indulge in behaviour that creates risk such as buying sex or injecting drugs. There is no doubt that economic power does create possibilities for engaging in safer behaviour; using the above-mentioned examples, this would mean capacity to buy and, thus, use condoms or to ascertain single use of needles and syringes. Whether safer behaviour is more possible due to improvement in one's economic situation may depend on other factors including what is socially accepted and culturally encouraged, educational status, and gender. It is necessary to recognize that the factors that affect vulnerability in the context of gender are not uniform across cultures and within different social segments, especially in terms of how they relate with other factors such as age and socio-economic background including education and earning capacity.

Education too has a Similar Impact

Data from studies in a few African countries, especially in the early years of the HIV epidemic, indicate that infection rates are at times higher among the more educated class, especially among men[5]. These findings indicate links between higher social status and opportunities for greater sexual contacts in some contexts. At the same time, in few of these African countries, young women with more education responded more favourably to HIV prevention efforts to promote safer sex. Such findings alarm us against over-simplification of the vulnerability paradigm. With regard to HIV/AIDS, the ultimate aim of risk and vulnerability reduction is to help people to exert control over their own risk by a process of individual and collective empowerment as well as to develop societal programmes that create an environment in which safer and protective behaviour can be practised.

Expanded Response to HIV/AIDS

Risk-reduction methods form the major constituent in HIV/ AIDS programmes since their inception. Clearly there in enough proof which exists to show that many such efforts do work and merit reinforcement . Successes in HIV prevention using the risk-reduction approach have been documented over the past few year[6,7]. These include programmes that target condom promotion, voluntary counselling and testing services, provision of information, needle and syringe exchange programmes, provision of STD diagnostic and treatment services, and containment of mother-to-child transmission. However, current programmes have several limitations. Some of them would benefit greatly from access to the best practices that have evolved from the worldwide effort respond to the epidemic. Often, programmes are not related to the changing needs of the communities for whom they are designed owing to lack of involvement of affected communities. Some also lack funds and thus cannot be taken to task. Interventions may also be undertaken individually, rather than in collaboration of each other. Where programmes work, it is important to give facts about what does and does not work, and what is the most efficient approach. An evidence-based approach can not only help to ascertain greater accountability and value for money, but also provide much for others to learn from.

So as to have a substantial impact on the epidemic, risk-reduction interventions must be rigorously designed according to best practices and adapted to local needs; they need to collect and share evidence of what makes them work and how. Such efforts, when successful, need to be expanded considerably, and reinforced worldwide. The strengthening of risk-reduction strategies thus forms a major dimension of expanding the response to HIV/AIDS.

Vulnerability Reduction Measures

The other aspect of expanding the response that complements risk-reduction effort is the reduction of vulnerability. Such efforts need to be targeted first within both. HIV/AIDS specific and other health-related programmes. Secondly, they need to be implemented within other sectors in order to bring about a multisectoral approach towards attaining the comparative advantages of these sectors where efforts will influence the spread of HIV. The cost of including HIV/AIDS in these broader programmes is often marginal. Vulnerability-reduction measures are in themselves necessary in the context of social justice and for overall development. However, in the context of HIV/AIDS. Such measures result in making an enabling and supportive environment for risk-reduction strategies to work. Vulnerability-reduction strategies in HIV/AIDS are based on the recognition of individual risk-taking behaviours, and of the personal and societal factors that affect them. Hence, an expanded response to HIV/AIDS becomes possible at several levels: minimises risks themselves through direct prevention, care and support and impact-alleviation efforts; and it influences vulnerability through social, cultural and economic change.

The latter approach of engaging sectors and partners not just to work for HIV/AIDS is not entirely new to many countries. However, until now, other than of some countries like Zambia, Uganda and Thailand, to name a few prominent examples, such a wide response has received neither sufficient attention nor funds. More so, in some cases, it has unfortunately amounted to the haphazard dispersion of HIV/AIDS activities within health and social programmes, with questionable impact on the epidemic.

In Zambia for instance, different ministries have made specific commitments to addressing HIV/AIDS. The Cabinet Office has set up HIV counselling services. The Office of the President has initiated the inclusion of HIV prevention messages in all speeches of the country's top political leaders. The Ministry of Defence has developed a plan for creating an orphans' fund to help with the maintenance and education of orphans of officers and men of the defence forces. The Ministry of Agriculture, Food and Fisheries proposes to train extension workers in social mobilization methods for HIV/AIDS prevention and care, and in coping mechanisms for rural populations. The Ministry of Local Government and Housing is examining land policies and establishing AIDS offices in all its units across Zambia. The Ministry of Tourism is incorporating HIV/AIDS into the syllabus of wildlife management schools and hotel and tourism managing institutes.

In Thailand the next five-year national AIDS plan will see how social and economic development can contribute to the control of HIV/AIDS, bringing HIV prevention and care efforts into the National Economic and Social Development Plan for 1997-2001. To care for people with AIDS, whose figures are expected to rise steadily for the next five years, increased funds will be needed. Here too, Thailand is taking a broad-based multisectoral approach. In addition to working to modify access to hospital medical care and treatment, community and family-based care approaches are being expanded, and efforts are under way to solve problems of social and economic support for and discrimination against those with HIV and AIDS. The Ministry of the Interior, which is incharge of community development, organizes training in non-discrimination and in basic family care for village headmen, housewives' organisations and youth groups. The Ministry of Education, which is in charge of Buddhist temples, promotes Buddhist teachings on compassion for monks, who then teach temple-goers. In some villages the Ministry helps the temples to house and look after indigent people with HIV. The Office of the Prime Minister, which is incharge of mass media, provides financing and secures corporate finance for messages on compassion, non-discrimination and family care through television, radio and newspapers, and encourages the private sector to incorporate these messages into their commercial advertisements.

If other sectors and partners are to join in the fight against this epidemic, they need to understand HIV/AIDS as a social and development issue and not just one of health. This understanding on the one hand needs planning, for the social, economic, political and indeed all development-related after effects of the epidemic so as to reduce its impact. On the other hand, it involves recognizing that social and development programmes themselves can in fact exacerbate the epidemic, and therefore, ascertain that appropriate measures are taken, especially in the case of those who are marginalized. To explain further, the construction of a major highway, the launching of a waterworks project, or the setting up of a free-trade zone necessitates consideration of the ways in which such activities may exacerbate the epidemic through disintegration of families, rapid urbanization, absence of familiar social-support systems or other consequences. It is necessary to implement measures to ascertain that these negative effects may be countered in order to reduce risks to populations affected.

While some factors of vulnerability reduction can be worked on in the short- or medium term through changes in law and policy, others will require a long process of cultural, structural and environmental changes in most societies. By setting medium-term and long-term goals for action targeted at vulnerability reduction, one can inculcate a manageable universe out of daunting and seemingly overwhelming challenges. This phased and multi-dimensional approach enables in handling the urgent needs of the epidemic, while simultaneously acting towards broader changes in society that will take time to bring about, but which are essential to any long-term impact on the epidemic.

Actions Aimed at Reducing Vulnerability

Actions aimed at reducing vulnerability in the short or medium term may include, for example: changing laws and policies that discriminate against specific populations; changing laws that increase risk, for example, by prohibiting payment of wages in bars or prohibiting alcohol sale during pay days, adding taxes on alcohol; and giving more attention to the needs of vulnerable populations like women in ongoing development schemes. They would also include ensuring that HIV/AIDS programmes are culturally suited, and increasing the reach of available services and programmes to vulnerable populations.

Long-term actions aimed at reducing vulnerability may include initiating cultural changes, specially with respect to the status of women. In the area of social norms and values, particularly with regard to sex. There object may be of bridging economic disparity through poverty-reduction policies and programmes. Also, they may work towards strengthening the overall capacity of health systems to fight against illness and death related to HIV/STD.

The Method of Expanding Response

Epidemiological, economic, social and behavioural data can be crucial to better understand the factors that increase vulnerability in any given society, as well as to identify where and how societal transformation is required. The relevance, quality and eventual impact of such vulnerability analysis will be increased by a broader participation, especially by those living with HIV/AIDS and affected individuals and communities, in the process of examining available information, sharing observations and designing the main avenues for focused action. Expansion of the response, however, neither means 'more of the same', nor initiates an unfocused approach; it does not even suggest more funds for

HIV/AIDS-specific efforts alone. What it does suggest is that best practices guide and influence the quality of the response; and that the response be more inclusive, such that the epidemic is taken into account while planning or implementing programmes in other sectors that are affected by and impacting on the HIV/AIDS epidemic. Such inclusiveness is more likely to be catalytic while strengthening the efforts of these sectors in the first place, as well as to integrate HIV/AIDS-specific activities better, so as to ascertain their long-term sustainability and effectiveness. It also brings new and untapped resources to bear on the epidemic.

A young woman for instance will benefit from sexual health education and access to services in diminishing her risk of acquiring HIV infection. In the medium term, such information and services aimed at vulnerability reduction need to be integrated in comprehensive adolescent health programmes that focus on sexual negotiation skills and empowerment of women. Vulnerability analysis may suggest that gender inequity in employment opportunity or income level puts this young woman and many others like her at a disadvantage, and reduces their potential to adopt safer behaviours. Vulnerability reduction requires short-term measures to increase women's economic self-reliance through alternative income-generating schemes and skill-building training programmes. Medium-term vulnerability reduction, on the contrary, calls for changes in labour laws and regulations, while long-term changes are needed in social norms and values related to gender equity and sex. The combined effect of the factors affecting this young women's risk and vulnerability may be further reduced through her participation in peer-support groups and other social support networks.

Expanding the global response to the epidemic thus includes strengthening risk-reduction efforts based on accumulated knowledge and innovations, combined with increasing those that aim at vulnerability reduction by creating a social and economic climate in which risk behaviour is likely to be reduced to the minimum. This process needs coordinated short-term and medium/long-term action by individuals and communities, as well as governments and private concerns, with the involvement of those living with and those affected by HIV/AIDS.

Routes to Expand the Response to HIV/AIDS

Expanding the response to HIV/AIDS may follow several paths. Few communities or nations will require to expand their response to HIV/AIDS in all these ways at one and the same time. Yet moving along only one of the routes to the neglect of others will not be sufficient for real expansion of the response. The need to prioritize and focus action remains crucial in this effort. Highlighting these pathways are the following principles:

(i) Analysis of factors that increase risk and vulnerability in order to develop a focused national strategy;

(ii) Widening of the quality and scope of HIV/AIDS strategies by identifying, promoting and applying best practice in short-term and long-term risk-reduction strategies and actions, and converting them to action; and

(iii) Increasing the response to include those strategies that focus on vulnerability through short-term and long-term measures, thereby

  (a) reaching vulnerable populations and focusing the socio-economic and cultural factors that influence vulnerability;

  (b) ascertaining that interventions and strategies support and complement each other to provide an umbrella of comprehensive and mutually reinforcing services;

  (c) reinforcing and introducing where required, evidence-based strategies for risk-reduction and continuing to monitor and improve them and disseminating the evidence.

This may include ascertaining best practices in information, education and the provision of prevention, care and support services; the replication of strategies that have proved successful; the design and implementation of new strategies according to evolving needs; the incorporation of HIV/AIDS work in other ongoing health and social programmes; the promotion and protection of the human rights of people living with HIV/AIDS; and targeting on those most vulnerable to HIV/AIDS in society.

Dimensions of Expanded Response to HIV/AIDS

An expanded response to HIV/AIDS may proceed in several dimensions:

(I) *Expanding coverage*, geographically and by population, by reaching out to marginalized communities in both urban and rural areas; demographically, by reaching out to women and men in the most sensitive age groups, especially young people and marginalized populations; and by addressing other factors that affect coverage for stigmatized and marginalized populations like sex workers and injecting drug users, with special attention to and finances for programmes serving mobile populations (migrants, displaced persons, refugees, and mobile occupations). A variety of innovative mechanisms need, to be used to reach some populations. For example in rural areas the services of companies marketing popular products could be utilised to distribute condoms to their distributing outlets,- young people may be communicated with better through media that are popular with the young and through young peoples' organisations.

(II) *Focusing action*, by directing public HIV finances in the first place to those who are most vulnerable to HIV infection, and are least likely to benefit from privately financed programmes for prevention, care and support.

(III) *Expanding collaboration in the design, implementation and evaluation of HIV/AIDS related policies and programmes* by enlisting the coordinated participation of governments, nongovernmental organisations, private sector, communities and individuals-especially, people living with and, affected by HIV/AIDS. Through local and affected communities one will have a better knowledge of factors influencing risk and vulnerability and to be able to recognize sustainable ways to address them. At the same time bringing in new partners that should be involved but have not been so, such as the private sector, is crucial. A multisectoral response is thus critical to an effective response to HIV/AIDS. The expansion of partnership in every element of the programme meals the sharing of responsibilities, mutual accountability, and effective coordination mechanisms.

(IV) *Involving all relevant sectors* by:

(a) promoting for and integrating HIV/AIDS containment and care into development initiatives and efforts;

(b) projecting and monitoring the effect of socio-economic development on people's vulnerability to HIV/AIDS;

(c) advocate impact-alleviation, providing support and care, and containing HIV as essential considerations for all socio-economic planning; and by

(d) utilizing the strengths of all sectors including religious groups, armed forces and such other groups.

Participation of all sectors of society and the economy in the response to HIV/AIDS should not just mean the inclusion of an HIV/AIDS project in a particular sector's work, but the analysis of sectoral factors that may effect people's risk-taking behaviours and vulnerability to HIV/AIDS, the sectoral contribution to reducing risk and vulnerability in these populations, and the accountability of these sectors in these areas.

(V) *Expanding finances mobilized in support of HIV/AIDS prevention and care* by mobilizing and making maximum use of available and diverse human, institutional and financial resources nationally and internationally, and by reinforcing resources not just for direct HIV/AIDS-related work but for all related socio-economic and health-related efforts. While all available finances, whether local, national or international, should be utilized more judiciously, efforts should also be made to towards skill-building in further mobilization of resources. These efforts will not only mitigate the spread and impact of HIV/AIDS, but will also reinforce the capacities of different sectors to become self-sufficient. In terms of resources this is not an impossible task. For instance, the incorporation of sex education into an existing school curriculum does not need additional funds and permits access to large numbers of young people.

(VI) *Increasing the sustainability of HIV/AIDS programmes over time* by reinforcing local and national self-reliance in the design and implementation of short-term and medium- or long-term initiatives and thereby building national capacity to do so. Renewed work towards community mobilization; decentralization of the responsibility of HIV/AIDS programmes, and delegation of authority and resources to the level that is nearest to the community; and more effective promotion for an expanded response to HIV/AIDS are all necessary to enhance the sustainability of the response to the epidemic.

All these dimensions need the exchange of knowledge and experience achieved in widening the response to the HIV/AIDS epidemic by sharing information locally, nationally and internationally, with stress on documenting the effectiveness and the impact of innovative approaches and on promoting evidence-based approaches. The design and application of effective monitoring, evaluation and research methods for an analysis of the epidemic — both its dynamics and its determinants — are equally essential if we are to draw lessons for shaping the response. The need for research on new technologies for prevention and care and on societal and behavioural interventions becomes all the more crucial for reinforcing an expanded response.

In sum of the global response to HIV/AIDS indicates that the paradigm being proposed is neither totally new and untested nor impossible to put into action, both from the perspective of public health in general and HIV/AIDS in particular. Many countries have already moved along the proposed dimensions to some degree: Thailand, Uganda and Zambia, to name a few. HIV/AIDS has multiple facets namely-biomedical, socio-economic, political, and cultural, and these provide strong arguments for the need for a multi-dimensional approach. Such a model includes two dimensions: persuasive, aiming at the individual for changes in risk behaviour, and enabling, as it is more directed at societal and contextual factors that allow and encourage safer behaviour in the context of HIV/AIDS and the lowering of vulnerability to HIV/AIDS. It also acknowledges the comparative advantages of different sectors in influencing the response and argues strongly for a sustainable response that empowers those affected by the epidemic. Few communities or countries - if any - will consider whether they will or will not require any further expansion their current response to the epidemic. The process of moving along the proposed dimensions, however needs to be advocated alongwith tools to put this into practice. The process of national strategic planning and review proposed by UNAIDS gives an opportunity to implement and monitor this expansion in the different directions, keeping in mind the broad principle of enhancing the quality and scope of the response*. Additional measures and tools may be developed as needed on the basis of experience gained over time in proceeding along these dimensions.

While arguing for expanding the response, UNAIDS acknowledges that many questions are likely to emerge. For instance, will the focus on vulnerability mean a neglect of the crucial needs of the epidemic to the benefit of those changes that are more difficult to bring about and which other sectors have been working towards for several years, often with little accomplishment? With the recent news of advances in treatment, is there really need to focus on those aspects of the epidemic that are more difficult to influence? Are the limited resources likely to be sufficient to address what appears to be an expanded agenda? Can we provide data to establish a direct linkage between influencing broader societal change and limiting the spread of the HIV/AIDS?

Some of these questions have been addressed, even if partially in this chapter. There will be additional questions that will continue to emerge. The world has to respond effectively and with brevity to what is a complex epidemic that demands a multi-dimensional and dynamic response. UNAIDS given priority to collecting evidence to show that such a response serves long-term needs while meeting the short-term ones, and that it is both ethically and technically sound.

* UNAIDS and its co-sponsors provide technical assistance to countries in national strategic planning along these lines. Modules that focus on specific aspects such as situation assessment, response review, strategic planning, and resource mobilization are available.

References

1. World Health Organization. *The Global AIDS Strategy*. WHO AIDS Series; 11, Geneva:WHO, 1992.
2. Mann J and Tarantola D. *"Introduction" in AIDS in the World II*, Oxford and New York: Oxford University Press, 1996.

3. Tawil O, Verster A and O'Reilly K. Enabling approaches for HIV/AIDS prevention: Can we modify the environment and minimize the risk? *AIDS*, 1995; 9: 1299-1306.
4. Reid E. *Placing Women at the Centre of the Analysis*. Issues Paper 6, HIV and Development Programme, UNDP, New York: UNDP, 1990.
5. *Confronting AIDS: Public Priorities in a Global Epidemic*. A World Bank Policy Research Report, Oxford & New York: Oxford University Press, 1997.
6. Aggleton P. *Success in HIV Prevention: Some Strategies and Approaches*. UK: AVERT, 1997.
7. HIV Prevention Works: Report of the Official Satellite Symposium, XIth International Conference on AIDS, Vancouver 1996.

Five

UNAIDS

Goal of UNAIDS India

UNAIDS India has made significant contributions in achieving its goals though its strategies and programs. It has enabled a common platform for the UN agencies the bilaterals, the govt. and the NGOs to work together. Presently, India is reported to have 3.86 million HIV infected people. Government of India is currently implementing the second phase of National AIDS Control Programme (NACP II). The main object of NACP II is to evolve a decentralized framework by giving more responsibility to State AIDS Control Societies (SACS).

Key constituents of this program are:

(a) Focused Intervention for communities at high risk;
(b) Containment of HIV transmission in populations at low risk;
(c) Reinforcing institutional strength;
(d) Providing low cost care, and
(e) Intersectoral linkages

The goal of UNAIDS India, a wing of its global mandate, is to catalyze, reinforce and orchestrate the unique skills, resources and networks of influence from other UN agencies and key-partners. Since its formation in 1996, it has been formulating its strategies and programs to meet the specific requirements of India. It has been playing a major role in enhancing Cosponsor involvement in fighting the epidemic and enabling a collaborative process between its stakeholders, namely, UN Cosponsor Agencies, the Government, bilateral agencies and civil society organisations including NGOs. UNAIDS has also played a key role in providing information and support. It has been actively assimilating best global practices on different issues and HIV-related interventions.

A major thrust has been to inspire Cosponsor agencies to priorities HIV in their program agenda.

UNAIDS has been giving substantial technical assistance to National AIDS Control Organisation (NACO) and the SACS, through its well designed innovative mechanisms, such as Virtual Teams, Theme Groups and Technical Resource Groups (TRGs). Priority areas where UN Agencies can intervene have also been identified. The effort throughout has been to evolve suitable models of interventions, which the government can then scale up across the country. For example, UNICEF has been actively supported in its current interventions on Mother-To-Child Transmission (MTCT). Specific work plans for each UN Agency and bilaterals are in place with clearly defined outputs.

An important objective of UNAIDS India has been to priorities HIV/AIDS on the national and state agenda. It has played a major role in sensitizing opinion leaders and policy makers on HIV/AIDS issues in an effort to place it as a development priority. A meeting of young parliamentarians with the Executive Director of UNAIDS, a video conference with Chief Ministers from three large states and talks with key political leaders, including the Prime Minister of India, have been the main components of this effort. UNAIDS has also been inspiring advocacy efforts for interventions by involving HIV/AIDS affected people, to make the programs more compliant and effective.

A key object purpose of developing collaborative network is to link external inputs with national priorities. With the National Programme working more successfully in consultation and collaboration with the UN System, Bilateral donors and Civil Society Organisations, UNAIDS is in the crucial position of reinforcing the collaborative efforts to these agencies in containing the HIV/AIDS epidemic. This also implies that enormous challenges will have to be faced and handled carefully. This would include the need to evolve new partners including the corporate sector. It calls for further advocacy with new members making new strategies and increasing the involvement of affected groups.

The Year 2000 has been a move in this direction by UNAIDS towards addressing these challenges. This study is an account of activities undertaken by UNAIDS during the year 2000. It attempts to provide a specific framework in which UNAIDS operates in India and to what extent it has been able to meet its objectives.

It also assesses the complex web of issues that make HIV/AIDS interventions an imminent challenges, notwithstanding the many positive efforts. And lastly, it tries to recognise the challenges that lie ahead for UNAIDS to continue fighting the epidemic with full force.

HIV/AIDS Prevalence in India

The threat posed by HIV/AIDS in India, in spite of interventions by government agencies as well as civil society organisations including NGOs, in the last 15 years, remain serious. The epidemic is one of the most serious public health problems in India. Occurrence of infection cases in all parts of the country reveals the spread from urban to rural areas and from high risk groups to the general population. Migration of labour, low literacy levels result in low awareness, gender disparities, occurrence of sexually transmitted diseases and reproductive tract infections are some of the factors responsible for this rapid spread. Found in India for the first time in 1986, now India is estimated to have 3.86 million HIV affected people at the end of year 2000. HIV infections have been reported from all States and union territories. Still driven largely by heterosexual transmission, HIV is spreading rapidly into the general population. The pattern of prevalence is now shifting towards women and young people with an simultaneous increase in vertical transmission and paediatric HIV.

With increase in gender disparities, the epidemic affects more and more women who end up bearing the brunt of its negative consequences. Women are now estimated to constitute nearly 25 per cent of new HIV infections. The inclination to stigmatize women in such situations worsens the problem further. The infection is also seen to be moving rapidly in the informal sector, which accounts for as much as 93 per cent of the workforce in India. Low productivity, poor living conditions, inadequate social protection and low levels of income are some of the factors that lead to this situation. HIV/AIDS goes beyond the issue of public health and raises fundamental question of human rights and threatens key development accomplishments in many areas. Protection of human rights is necessary to safeguard human dignity. When rights are protected, fewer people get infected, and those living with HIV/AIDS as well as their families can deal better with the disease. The complexity of the problem is being stressed because of its impact on the entire spectrum - societies, communities, families and individuals. This has led to a whole range of question regarding social and health care support.

The rise in AIDS cases is diminishing the ability of families and communities to support and care for their children, resulting in new problems. Today, the burden of AIDS is becoming increasingly evident. The epidemic is in a fairly advanced stage in Maharashtra, Tamil Nadu and Manipur. In Maharashtra, for instance, 60 per cent of sex workers tested were found to be infected. HIV has reached 14-60 per cent in Sentinel STD Clinics and is found in over 2 per cent of women attending antenatal clinics. Since the problem in these States was found early, it is becoming more evident. Of the total bed occupancy in Imphal and Mumbai hospitals, HIV associated illnesses account for 24-40 per cent cases.

In the past 4 years, the epidemic has spread fast across other southern and western states, as well as in the North East which has a high prevalence of HIV among injecting drug users.

Because of the sharp increase of HIV infections in Andhra Pradesh and Karnataka, these two states have gone ahead of Tamil Nadu. While HIV prevalence is still low in many other states the occurrence of high levels of Sexually Transmitted Diseases (STDs) along with the presence of sexual networks and migration make of high vulnerability imminent. A study, conducted in 1999, has revealed that injecting drug use is on the rise; nearly 45 per cent of attendees, linked to an IDU treatment centre in New Delhi, tested positive[1]. Although the epidemic has moved far beyond its initial estimates on people engaging themselves in risk behaviour, trends of sub-epidemics are becoming more than visible in these very groups. The need to closely monitor this pattern amongst commercial sex workers (CSWs) or injecting drug users (IDUs) and men having sex with men (MSM), is urgent because of the implications it has for a wider heterosexual epidemic. Based on these epidemiological findings, the program has been focused on preventive strategies in states with low prevalence of HIV, while the dual strategy of prevention and control will be implemented in the states with high prevalence of HIV.

Indian Government's Response to HIV/AIDS

India is one of the few countries where HIV prevention activities were begun at a very initial stage of the epidemic. Government response to the problem was as early as in 1986 and the National AIDS Control Organisation (NACO) was set up in 1991. Phase I of the program was initiated with the assistance of the World Bank. NACO was formed within the Ministry of Health and Family Welfare with a senior IAS official, of the rank of Additional Secretary to the Government of India, to enable quick decision making. The setting up of NACO saw many accomplishments, including an increased level of awareness, setting up of infrastructure at the state level for programme implementation and modifications in blood safety. However, there was an evident requirement to create a sense of ownership amongst states, particularly by involving NGOs in the program. The emphasis of the program tended to be medical - a health issue, with the need to focus on social and developmental implications.

Characteristics of the Epidemic in India

(a) The mode of transmission in India is heterosexual in more than 90 per cent of cases.
(b) The 15-49 year age group has the highest prevalence of STDs and HIV infection.
(c) The probability of STD patients getting infected by HIV is 5-10 times more than among those without STDs.
(d) State epidemics can be categorized as generalised, concentrated and low, based on the following definitions:
   (i) *Generalised:* States where HIV prevalence is 1 per cent or more in antenatal women.
   (ii) *Concentrated:* Where HIV prevalence in antenatal women in less than 1 per cent while the prevalence in STD and other high-risk groups is 5 per cent more.
   (iii) *Low:* States where the HIV prevalence in antenatal women is less than 1 per cent while the prevalence in STD and other high risk groups is less than 5 per cent.

Based on the lessons learnt in Phase I of the program, the current Phase II response has adopted a twin approach. While it is evident that groups with high-risk behaviour cannot be ignored, it is also vital to adopt a multi-sectorial approach. The current phase of the National Program sees a more de-centralised approach and building up capacities at state level, with the states taking on larger responsibilities for implementation.

NACO has launched State AIDS Control Societies (SACS) with mechanisms for program management at the state level. Each state has designed a Program Implementation Plan (PIP) which is based on extensive consultations with different sectors in the state including NGOs, community groups and different Ministries. SACS include a strong NGO constituent on targeted interventions and community mobilization on STD/RTIs. In the last two years, there has been a major endeavour towards supporting the state programs by mobilizing technical resources within the country, specially with the setting up of Technical Resource Groups (TRGs). Surveillance has also been increased. Issues of Care and Support, comprising of home based care and continuum of care has been taken up as an important component of the National AIDS Prevention Policy. Some steps taken in this direction are: voluntary blood-testing centres, drugs for management of opportunistic infections and setting up of more counseling centres.

Objectives for the Year 2000

Working alongwith NACO, the Theme Group set itself the following target areas for the year 2000:

(a) Support greater development of collaborative framework;
(b) Support and reinforce TRGs;
(c) Support building of state capacities;
(d) Enable formation of Theme Group;
(e) Work within Human Rights framework;

UNAIDS Program Planning

In August 2000, the second UNAIDS strategic planning retreat was held in Bangalore. The first retreat was held in 1999. These retreats facilitated in planning a concerted effort in defining roles and responsibilities of collaborating agencies comprising the UN System, the Government and bilateral donors. The retreats have played an important part facilitating the UN agencies to develop strategies in their own areas of strength, which could be taken to scale by the National Program. The Bangalore retreat addressed questions central to the current stage of the national response to the epidemic. Important topic for discussion that were identified here included[2].

(i) Making decentralization a reality;
(ii) Building stronger partnerships at the state level;
(iii) Addressing Stigma; and
(iv) Growing concern on the IDU problem in the North East.

Organized jointly by UNAIDS and NACO, the retreat emphasized on the implementation of phase II of the National Program. With emphasis on decentralization, focus was on planning interventions in the states, building capacities at state level and addressing the question of absorptive capacities.

Attention

Five major areas of challenge were also identified. These were:

(a) Need to build capacities within state;
(b) Ensuring that targeted interventions achieve desired impact;
(c) Achieving behaviour change outside the "High-Risk" populations;
(d) Need to face discrimination and stigma;
(e) Addressing the need of care and support

Strategy meeting have helped highlight the overall national strategy and gaps that UNAIDS, as a support organisation, can address. The strategic planning retreat was followed by Theme Group meetings. These meetings have been crucial in defining the role expectations from UNAIDS by stakeholder institutions. This also led to the formulation of a work plan for UNAIDS.

UN Response of HIV/AIDS

(a) The UN system has the mission of enabling a multisectoral response to HIV with the help of joint programming.

(b) The UN system facilitates active involvement of NACO and bilaterals in the Theme Group which is the premier body governing UN response in India.

The UN system has many innate strengths owing to its structure and global mandate. UN agencies have close working relationships with the Government through different ministries and departments and thereby have scope of engaging in policy dialogue. It has partnerships with civil society which provide for grassroot experiences and learning. Thus, the UN system is unparalleled in addressing a mandate that cuts across a range of key issues such as gender and human rights, health, poverty reduction and broad development strategies. It supports government efforts to inculcate partnerships with all representatives of civil society. However, since resources to fight HIV/AIDS epidemic are usually limited, UN Agencies leverage these advantages to initiate focussed and well defined areas of contribution, falling within the mandate of each agency. Some of these strategies involve developing partnerships around HIV with ministries and civil society; mainstreaming HIV within their own agency programmes; supporting attempts in mainstreaming human rights, gender and approaches to poverty eradication.

UNAIDS: The Beginning

Till 1986, World Health Organisation (WHO) was the UN Agency which had undertaken the lead role and responsibility on AIDS through the Global program on AIDS (GPA). But the rapid spread of the infection by mid-90s made clear the need for a more focused and expanded UN effort beyond health to tackle the serious consequences on human lives. It was also evident that it would be difficult for one UN agency to take on the mandate of addressing the HIV/AIDS epidemic. The need for greater coordination in an attempt to maximise the impact was felt. So as to meet this challenge, the United Nations employed an innovative approach in 1996 by making six organisations collaborate in a joint and cosponsored programme - the Joint United Nations Programme on HIV/AIDS or UNAIDS. The six original cosponsors of UNAIDS-UNICEF, UNDP, UNFPA, UNESCO, WHO, and the World Bank — were joined by UNDCP in 1999. Working on the same platform through UNAIDS, the cosponsors expand their outreach with other UN Agencies, with the Governments, with Civil Society Organisations and regional and country level networks of people living with AIDS.

UNAIDS in India

UNAIDS in India performs four major functions:

(a) Coordination of the UN system's HIV/AIDS response;
(b) Advocacy;
(c) Building/strengthening partnerships; and
(d) Providing information

The goal of the organisation, under the larger umbrella of its global mandate, is to catalyze, reinforce and orchestrate the unique skills resources and networks of influence from other UN agencies. Its uniqueness lies in the fact that it is a co-sponsored institution, within the UN system, created specifically and exclusively to respond to the HIV epidemic. It enables co-sponsor engagement in significant areas suited to the Indian needs. UNAIDS co-sponsors from among the UN System are: UNICEF, UNDP, UNFPA, UNESCO, UNDCP, WHO and the World Bank. Other UN agencies actively working in the Indian UN Theme Group comprise of ILO and UNIFEM. In addition, bilateral agencies such as DFID, USAID, CIDA, SIDA and AUSAID have given the program firm and committed support through participation in the Theme Group.

Off late, there has been a greater stress on decentralization and better inter-institutional coordination. In working together, the Agencies have been able to expand and reinforce their network through strategic alliances with other UN Agencies, Bilateral Agencies, regional and country networks of people living with HIV/AIDS and other Non-governmental Organisations (NGOs).

To work according to its global mandate of addressing AIDS by ploughing back lessons from the countries in which it is engaged, UNAIDS India has designed its global strategies to specific socio-economic needs of India. These strategies depend on several factors such as the Government response to the problem, its policies, economic situation, and so on. These are also based on social factors, values and norms that are prevalent at a point of time. To some extent, they are based on the response of other agencies working on the issue. The response of the civil society organisations, for instance, is well acknowledged in addressing the issue of HIV/AIDS. The UNAIDS India has set its goals and objectives keeping these factors in mind. The task at hand involves keeping in account the resources available. The roles have been decided by taking into account co-sponsor requirements as well.

UNAIDS - Key Roles

(1) Coordination: Coordinated UN System response
(2) Advocacy: Advocacy for enhanced political and policy support
(3) Building/Strengthening Partnerships:
   (a) Strategic Planning/Technical Assistance for multisectoral responses
   (b) Coordinate and build community/civil society responses
(4) Knowledge Management:
   (a) Catalyse technical support processes at state level
   (b) Strengthen Technical Resource Network in the country, and UNAIDS role as knowledge centre.
   (c) Respond to emerging issues

UNAIDS India: Key Roles

In keeping with the broader mandate of UNAIDS and the response to the epidemic in India, UNAIDS in India identified the following roles[3]:

(a) Coordination: For the complete UN System, extended to other bilateral agencies
(b) Support: For National HIV/AIDS Program
(c) Service: For different co-sponsors and stakeholders by giving information, best practices, for instance, and providing technical inputs, such as a monitoring and evaluation framework
(d) Institutional Capacity Building: For local level organisations, at the national and state level related to programme planning and implementation
(e) Advocacy: Impacting socio-political perspectives on how the epidemic is viewed in India

Although these roles are connected to each other, they have different constituencies and call for careful planning to ensure effective implementation.

The Structure of UNAIDS Network

The challenge for UNAIDS lies in the fact that it works within a gamut of institutions. UNAIDS India has several stakeholders who are its constituencies. The organisation works in close association with other Agencies in the UN System, with the National Program, with bilaterals, with SACS and civil society organisations. These institutions, about from being the stakeholders of UNAIDS: also have their own structure, agenda and programs. They work on their commitment to the epidemic through their own programs and resources. From UNAIDS, they seek additional role to arrive at their common objectives. The organisation has initiated institutional mechanisms to enhance its major roles of support and coordination. The endeavour has been to avoid a large and vertical program structure. Some of these innovations include setting up of an inter-institutional Theme Group, a Virtual Team (VT) of specialists in different UN Organisations and Technical Resource Groups (TRGs), which are created to provide technical support to the National Program on a comprehensive set of issues related to HIV/AIDS.

The cosponsors have identified two roles specifically for UNAIDS India:

(a) Assisting in the capacity building process of NACO and the SACS comprising of the development of and assistance in formulating a strong monitoring and evaluation system for the National Program.

(b) Be a technical group that can ascertain dissemination of global best practices and ascertain that they be adopted within the National Program.

Coordinated UN System Response

An important objective of UNAIDS India has been to enable greater cosponsor involvement in the program. The strategy has been to strengthen the Theme Group process and support the co-sponsors in developing their own work plans. UNAIDS assisted this process with the help of its secretariat which ascertains effective outputs from each Theme Group meeting. The Theme Group met thrice in the year and gave strategic directions to the National program. This year, ILO also joined the Theme group. Focal points on HIV, within each agency, have also been meeting regularly. Individual agencies have made important staff sensitization efforts for HIV/AIDS.

Setting up of Theme Group

The Theme Group began in 1998 and has since played an important role in guiding the activities of the secretariat. It has been strengthened with the involvement of co-sponsors, bilateral partners and the government. The Theme Group meets thrice a year to review progress and plays a crucial monitoring role for the secretariat and co-sponsor involvement. The Theme Group decides on priorities and the plan of action of the secretariat. The emphasis in the year 2000 was on operationalising the workplans that were developed by co-sponsors. These workplans have been finalized after a review by the Theme Group. The plan to operationalise was further reinforced with the formation of the virtual Team.

Formulation of the Virtual Team

One of the support mechanisms started by UNAIDS to deliver outputs/inputs from co-sponsors into the National response is the Virtual Team (VT). The UNAIDS secretariat plays a key enabling role in supporting the UN Co-sponsors in highlighting HIV in their work. This has been planned through the Virtual Team members. The Virtual Team has been in place and functional from the year 2000.

Objectives

To reinforce the multi-sectored responses to HIV/AIDS on national and state levels, using agency skills and promotion of counterpart collaboration.

So far, the Virtual Teams have been working mainly within the programs of their agencies. A major role that has been added to the Virtual Team is that of providing support at state level. Thus, the VT is placed in a strategic position to carry out support at state level so that the policy decisions at Theme Group level can be directly discussed with the states and can be supported during implementation. The main force behind this activity is the needs of the states. The key factor in the chance for strengthening state responses lies in the fact that:

(a) NACO has invited the Virtual Team to give support at state level, and
(b) The states have been demanding technical support on various issues

VT's Functions at State Level

(a) Strengthening multi-sectored response/partnerships
(b) Garnering resources
(c) Bridging the gap between TRGs and state technical resources
(d) Being a resource for strategic planning
(e) Identification and documentation of best practices
(f) Linking (demand creation) between TRGs and the states

As of now the Virtual Team consists of three different member categories that have different roles and functions in their support to the National Response. All Virtual Teams meet regularly, enabling information sharing and co-ordination. They follow strategies suited to their multiple modes of functioning.

A document which clearly demarcates VT strategies, state linkages, strengths and goals has now been finalised by the Theme Group.

The Virtual Team leader is the UNAIDS India Country Programme Adviser, who leads the team in close co-operation with the Project Director, NACO. In spite of being a new venture, the Virtual Team brings with it a range of issues and program-related skills which include: women's skill, youth program, issues related to drug abuse, focused interventions, communication and program-related experience and expertise.

UNAIDS Core Virtual Team

Agency	*Focus*
UNIFEM	Gender
UNICEF	Children, Youth, MTCT, Communication
UNDP	Development, Civil Society Response
UNESCO	Education
UNDCP	Drug Demand Reduction
WHO	Epidemiology, MTCT
ILO	Workplace Initiatives
UNAIDS	TI, VT Programme Support and Stakeholder Management, Strategic Planning, Law and Ethics

UNAIDS India: Review and Strategy

UNAIDS India carried out an internal review of the organisation's achievements and expectations. This review gave an opportunity for UNAIDS to review its roles, opportunities, strengths and weaknesses, both with respect to internal strategies as well as expectations of the stakeholders. The review also proposed restructuring and redesigning of some of the innovations so as to further strengthen the processes that are already operational. One such restructuring has been done with some of the TRGs.

Sensitization of the UN Staff

As a first step towards mainstreaming HIV, a series of sensitization workshops were held by UNICEF UNFPA and UNDP for their staff members. Due to which some of the staff members have initiated a dialogue with their programme partners to identify HIV-related issues and their effect on the related sectors.

Capacity Building for the States

With the emphasis on decentralization gaining importance, UNAIDS enabled a process of focussed and need-based capacity building for the states. The states got more support in program planning and implementation. The need to support SACS by accurate strategic planning was given major importance. Part of this capacity building exercise also meant designing state-appropriate Targeted Interventions (TI). For achieving this, the TRG on TIs was strengthened and other agencies such as NGOs and CBOs were also included in this process. So as to ascertain some degree of accountability and quality control, UNAIDS supported NACO in designing a Monitoring and Evaluation framework based on global observation as well as local needs. As a part of this, monitoring tools were developed. UNAIDS also developed tools for strategic planning. In line with this a TI manual has been developed and field-tested. It is now available as a best practice tool. All officials (nearly 120) of SACS were trained on TI planning. A TI consultant has also been appointed to support NACO. State AIDS Societies are given power to provide funding support to NGOs for targeted interventions. Program

Implementation Plans (PIPs) developed by the states in preparation for Phase II, provided a framework for starting up the activities. A working group on M&E has been established and consists of representatives from NACO, UNAIDS, DFID, USAID and the World Bank. UNAIDS supported the development of the M&E framework including Behavioural Sentinel Surveillance (BSS) and providing the tools for monitoring. The M&E framework is being executed in collaboration with the global indicators group at Laussane University, MERG and UNAIDS headquarters. The monitoring and evaluation framework has been developed jointly to ensure greater program coordination, efficiency and efficacy.

NACO and Targeted Interventions

The basic aim of Targeted Interventions is to decrease the rate of transmission amongst the most sensitive and marginalised sections of society. As one of the most important components of Phase II of the National Program, TI envisages a comprehensive and integrated strategy for addressing these groups in an effort to reduce their vulnerabilities and mitigate the impact of HIV/AIDS, thereby preventing the disease from spreading further. Targeted Interventions provide a basis for comprehensive intervention in marginal groups.

Development of National Technical Resource Networks

One of the significant interventions supported by UNAIDS has ben the development of a sustainable technical support network and efforts to build long term capacities in the country for strengthening state capacities.

Technical Resource Groups (TRGs)

TRGs were initiated to provide technical support to state programs/SACS through improved program design, by providing state-of-the-art knowledge in technical areas, by transferring the know-how to improve program implementation and by identifying best practices. The TRG initiative gathered momentum in the year 2000. UNAIDS supported strengthening of systems for TRG-State links by playing a major role in facilitating linkages between the National Program, state level programs as well as TRGs. So as to facilitate the transition towards a more state driven program, UNAIDS supported NACO in establishing systems for connectivity and TRG management. Following thus a TRG Management Cell was set up in NACO, with two senior scientists appointed to enable TRG-State linkages and peer review of best practices.

Thematic Area

For providing technical support to states, TRGs have been constituted, each covering a different thematic area: Clinical Management, Research and Development on HIV/AIDS, Counselling, STD, Women, Children and AIDS, Targeted Interventions, IDUs, Law and Ethics, Blood safety and Surveillance.

TRGs were reconstituted to demonstrate state's needs, based on a Technical Needs Assessment in three states. All the TRG Chairs, members and SACS were connected electronically and trained in Information Technology. AT the Bangalore Retreat, UNAIDS gave a hands-on interactive session on the Internet, thus linking up on-line with the NACO information center, to which 35 State AIDS Societies, all TRGs, UNAIDS and their co-sponsors are linked up. As a result of this, discussions on program themes are now weekly events led by NACO. These link-ups between TRG members and SACS have undoubtedly made communication faster and effective. Having finalized their workplans now, the TRGs have a state-of-the-art paper and several of them have been invited by SACS to provide technical assistance.

The year 2000 saw the launch of the portal site, youandaids.org. IT applications function under this umbrella. The portal enables a discussion forum for women, youth, positive people, chat groups, common massaging system, MIS linkages with Geographical Information System (GIS) and e-surveillance. A one-day training workshop on connectivity was also held. The portal has modified information exchange at all levels. UNAIDS has enabled the sharing of best practices by developing TRG-global network linkages. It has developed global and national best practices guides, strategies in partnership with NACO, TRGs, SACS and the UNAIDS headquarters. UNAIDS has also ascertained the dissemination of these global best practices.

Reduced Discrimination and Stigma

> "Discrimination against, and stigmatization of, HIV-infected people and people with AIDS and population groups, undermine public health and must be avoided."
>
> —*The London Declaration on AIDS, January, 1998.*

Social perception of fear, denial and stigmatization have since been long obstacles in countering the HIV epidemic in India, just like in many other parts of the world. This has had serious consequences on prevention programs and more importantly undermined the ability of individuals and societies to protect themselves and provide support and reassurance to those infected[4].

UNAIDS in India has made tackling stigma and discrimination a priority issue. In the Bangalore retreat on strategic planning, stigma was one of the main issues discussed. Presentations on the complexity of the issue highlighted the need for all partners to come together in tackling the issue.

Involving People Living With AIDS (PLWAs)

UNAIDS India has been making serious attempts to keep in step with the global mandate of ascertaining greater involvement of people with AIDS. The effort has been to encourage meaningful Greater Involvement of People with HIV/AIDS (GIPA) initiatives amongst all of its collaborators - governments, private sector, bilaterals and community partners. At the strategic planning retreat in the year 2000, positive peoples networks reinforced the need to create an enabling environment where widespread discrimination could be curbed by removing the veil of ignorance around HIV and PLWAs. This would inspire HIV counselling, testing, treatment and opportunities for positive people to be absorbed into the folds of society. Following proposal were made at the retreat:

(a) Urgent need for setting up workshops for media orientation to HIV issues and involving cable networks and regional print media as well.

(b) Sensitizing private and public health systems through cooperation with positive people.

(c) Including HIV positive national level UN volunteers in lecture tours around the country, for giving HIV a 'face' and de-stigmatizing the issue.

Alongwith these proposals meeting involving positive groups, media and communication agencies were also organized. Presentations were made by different groups on intervention experiences in India. Workshops on sensitization of the judiciary were also held. Another initiative has been the Photo-documentation 'People Plus' initiated by INP + networks. An exhibition of these photographs was held on World AIDS day. UNAIDS supported a National NGO convention which assembled NGOs from all over the country and helped identify their role within the National programme. It provided a platform for dialogue with the basic goal of supporting and strengthening the formation of networks of PLWAs, NGOs, CBOs and MSM.

National Conference on Human Rights and HIV/AIDS (2000)

For developing and reinforcing the response within the human rights framework, UNAIDS collaborated on a joint project on advocacy with the National Human Rights Commission (NHRC) this year. This first 'National Conference on Human Rights and HIV/AIDS' took place in New Delhi, in November 2000. The conference aimed at bringing about a dialogue between concerned agencies and groups on the connection between Human Rights and HIV/AIDS prevention and management. Organised by National Human Rights Commission (NHRC), together with National AIDS Control Organisation (NACO), Lawyers Collective, UNICEF and UNAIDS, the conference was the meeting point of major stakeholders including the NHRC, law enforcement agencies and NACO to identify key issues and prescribe an action plan.

The *objectives* of the conference were to:

(a) discuss and identify important issues in the HIV/AIDS related Human Rights framework;
(b) build connectivity between State Human Rights Commissions and the State AIDS Control Societies;
(c) identify future interventions to initiate an enabling environment at various levels; and
(d) identify steps to expand the response within a rights based strategy.

The conference was part of a series of meetings planned by the Core Group on Human Rights and Public Health established by

NHRC. It provided a forum and force to examine the role of Human Rights in its response to HIV/AIDS. It gave all partners the opportunity to view the importance of recognising, promoting and protecting Human Rights, implementing a sustainable environment and recognising the central role of law as necessary part of the response strategies to prevent and manage HIV/AIDS in India.

Working with Marginalised Groups

In an attempt to strengthen marginalised groups and in building their capacities to mainstream HIV, UNAIDS India supported to setting up of a National Sex Workers Forum. A strategic plan addressing issues of stigma and discrimination was also chalked out computer. MSM networks were supported in locating networks of community-based groups and their strategic needs. This, in turn, initiated development of technical support systems.

Promoting Behaviour Change Beyond the 'High Risk' Groups

The key approach to strengthen behaviour change beyond high-risk groups has been to address people at risk by broadbasing the response and streamlining HIV into the existing structures such as the local self government. While Phase II of the National Program has emphasized on targeted interventions, there is also an urgent requirement to address the bridge populations in the Indian setting. The Government is now focussing more emphatically on young people and migrant groups. Non-commercial sex is now seen as an important source of infection with 50 per cent of all new infections occurring in the age group of less than 25 years[5].

The effort has been to strengthen people to protect themselves. Innovative methods were employed to reach the population at large.

Family Health Awareness Week

UNAIDS supported NACO's endeavours at community mobilization through the Family Health Awareness Week. Set up with the idea of increasing awareness among and reaching out to communities at large, a third round of the FHAW took place in the first and second week of June 2000, across the country. The population estimated to be covered by the campaign is estimated to be 600 million, of which 34 million attended the Camps.[6].

The *objective* of Family Health Awareness Week which was initiated by NACO in 1999 were as follows:

(a) Bringing about awareness of HIV/AIDS and other STIs by involving the Primary Health Care structure

(b) Early detection and treatment of Reproductive Tract infections (RTIs)

Medical Officers and para-medical staff were trained in the selected 100 districts where the program was to be piloted. The training facilitated detection of STI cases and referring them to PHCs. The FHAW program was inspiring as large number of people came to several of these centres seeking treatment for RTIs and STIs in spite of initial apprehension. It also increased the possibilities of enhancing the awareness program among rural communities and facilitated better access to health care. It was an important step in generating a firm linkage between NACP and the primary health care centres, thereby encouraging the decentralization approach. UNAIDS and co-sponsors actively supported this endeavour of NACO. It is suggested that FHAW experiences and lessons for community involvement be documented as best practices in the Indian context.

Working with the Young

Of the globally-estimated 16,000 new infections daily, about 1,600 include children under the age of 15 years. Young people between the ages of 10 and 24 account for more than 50 per cent of new post-infancy infections all over the world. Investing in HIV prevention among young people is likely to contribute significantly to a more sustainable response to HIV/AIDS[7].

Moverover, the vulnerability of the youth to the infection becomes more severe due to several changing norms of the society. More and more young people are being recognized as a resource for changing the course of the epidemic. They are influenced by the HIV prevention programs and are effective promoters of HIV prevention action. As a result, UNAIDS has supported early interventions by focussing on adolescents with information on HIV/AIDS and the skills to improve their self confidence so that they can make effective decisions. They have enabled the formation of an inter-agency group for the development and piloting of a strategy for young people and out-of-the-school youth. This working group consizes of Representatives from UNICEF, UNESCO and UNFPA, UNICEF has also taken out adolescent health and education guidelines along with NACO.

Interventions at the Workplace

UNAIDS is initiating the development of a policy on non-discrimination at the workplace. In its planning phase, the project is a tripartite response to HIV intervention at the workplace. The project will be implemented by ILO in the coming year in close collaboration with UNAIDS, in full consultation with members of the Theme Group on HIV/AIDS in India. The project aims at initiating activities which would be systemic, cost-effective and properly aimed to mobilize the world of work for prevention of HIV/AIDS across the country.

Working with Panchayats

The year 2000 saw several innovative endeavours in reaching out to the general population, right up to the village level through the existing democratic institutions such as the 'Panchayats' or local governments. UNDP has been working for strengthening local self governments in an attempt to involve them in responding to the epidemic.

This also follows in with the decentralization efforts of the Government in the Phase II of the National Program. Local self governments, municipalities as well as Zila Parishads have been involved in this program. The aim of the program is to strengthen local initiatives and provide an enabling environment for alleviating stigma and discrimination.

The first round of sensitization took place in Tamil Nadu in the Gandhigram Rural Institute. Meetings were also held in Udupi and Gulbarga districts of Karnataka.

Advocacy

An important goal of UNAIDS India is to put HIV/AIDS as a priority issue on the national and state agenda. It has played a crucial role in sensitizing opinion leaders and policy makers on HIV/AIDS issues in an attempt to place it as a development priority. Given the changing socio-political circumstances, the current advocacy efforts were reinforced with policy makers. International exposure and interaction has led to greater political support to the program.

Political Advocacy

At the level of policy and political support, there has been a change in the momentum at both the highest level and in the states which are undergoing the most extensive spread of the epidemic. Political advocacy gained force with the Prime Minister of India urging Parliamentarians, in December 1998, to accept the existing situation as a challenge to India's development rather than only a health issue. Chief Ministers from many states have taken interest in mobilising their administration and in bringing about public awareness. For keeping up the momentum, UNAIDS has approached policy makers for controlling the epidemic. A meeting of 25 young Parliamentarians with the UNAIDS Executive Director, Dr. Peter Piots, in March 2000, was a platform for key political leaders to address issues of HIV. The team consisting of the Executive Director and the Country Program Advisor of UNAIDS, discussed with Parliamentarians the part they could play in controlling the epidemic. During the discussion, it was advised that the Parliamentarians could take the issue to their constituencies and focus on key people involved in local governance who, in turn, could communicate with the Members of Parliament in the area, with an endeavour to draw a political commitment from them. Members from various political parties of India, namely, Bhartiya Janta Party (BJP), Congress, CPI-M and DMK were present at this meeting. Although the meeting generated an eager response, the group members also voiced their apprehensions.

Issues of how to discuss sexuality or condom use in a public domain, and of the moving prospect of caring for children orphaned by AIDS - affected parents, were discussed. The meeting had an inspiring response. Several MPs showed interest in carrying the issue forward. Some of them, for instance in Sivaganga District of Tamil Nadu, even organized meetings at the Zila Parishad level in their own constituencies. The initial success resulted in more meetings with Chief Ministers and a video conference between CMs of three States - Maharashtra, Tamil Nadu and Andhra Pradesh (states with high prevalence) - and the Union Minister of Health, Dr Thakur, in November 2000. All the leaders in the conference agreed for a need to break the "silence". They also made commitments and suggestions of national significance. Some of the questions raised in the conference were related to: trafficking, introduction of sex education in schools, and the need to raise the issues at a political level. A meeting with leaders at the national level also led to more advocacy with political leaders across the country. Several discussions and video conferences have followed these endeavours. Meetings and discussions held with CMs from 10 states on HIV/AIDS have led to their including HIV in their political agenda. A 12-member team of program managers and policy makers also visited Uganda and key lessons were reflected in the state responses[8].

UNAIDS has also developed and distributed advocacy tools to influence policy makers and program implementers on the impact of HIV on development goals. A multimedia presentation kit on the AIDS epidemic in India has also been developed.

Sensitizing Policy Makers on Issues of Mother-to-Child Transmission[9]

There are around 12 million women of childbearing age all over the world who are HIV-positive. The number of infants who acquire the virus from their mothers is increasing rapidly in a number of places, including India and Southeast Asia. Mother-to-Child transmission (MTCT) is, by far, the biggest source of HIV infection in children below the age of 15 years[10]. NACO and UNICEF have been collaborating on the MTCT issue. UNAIDS supported this initiative of UNICEF in sensitizing the policy makers on the requirement for MTCT prevention.

Greater Involvement of Men

India, for the first time in the global south region launched a global theme on the World AIDS Day, 2000. The theme of "Greater Male Involvement" helped identifying crucial issues and strategies for male involvement and gave an opportunity for public debate and discussions on the issue. The theme was also chosen in an effort to encourage participation by men in adopting safer behaviours and playing a larger role in caring.

Why Focus on Men?

Five reasons for focussing the World AIDS Day Campaign on men are:

(a) Men's health is important but receives less attention;
(b) Men's behaviour exposes them to risk of HIV;
(c) Men's behaviour exposes women to risk of HIV;
(d) Unprotected sex between men endangers both men and women; and
(e) Men need to give greater thought to AIDS as it affects their families directly.

—*Reference: Men and AIDS a Gendered Approach, 2000 World AIDS Campaign, UNAIDS, Geneva*

The campaign had three main objects:

(a) Raise awareness of the relationship of men's behaviour and HIV.
(b) Encourage men and adolescent boys to make a commitment to help containment of HIV infection.
(c) Promote programs that address the needs of both men and women.

Coalition with the Corporate Sector

UNAIDS has been involved in the process of strengthening and sensitizing the corporate sector towards the cause of HIV/AIDS and has actively advocated the need for interventions in the workplace. The Theme Group has bee actively involved in supporting the issue. A meeting was organized with officials from the corporate sector and the Prime Minister's Office after which in a meeting with key business leaders, the Prime Minister of India called for the setting up of a business coalition on World AIDS Day.

International Day For Eradication of Poverty

Every year, 17th October is celebrated as the International Day for Eradication of Poverty by UNDP. The theme for the year,

2000 was "HIV/AIDS-Breaking the Silence". UNDP and UNAIDS jointly held a short commemorative event to re-examining and rededicate efforts towards poverty alleviation programmes and to focus on the link between HIV/AIDS and issues of poverty. For generating public interest, activities like street plays and talks were included. AIDS activists, working closely with HIV positive people spoke to the people gathered at the function.

Need for Care and Support

An increase in the number of people living with HIV has created the need to provide adequate care and support, both medical and social. With limited treatment facilities and no cure available, India could face a crisis with serious after effects on the productive human resource.

The Government recognizes the need to provide care and support that is suitable and feasible. Providing for these needs in circumstances where resources are restricted and the numbers are large is a challenging. Alongwith its lead partners, WHO and the International Alliance on HIV/AIDS, UNAIDS has prepared a strategy paper on care and support. Work has begun in collaboration with UNCTAD on compulsory licensing of HIV drugs in India. In a preliminary meeting, UNAIDS invited officials from the Ministry of Commerce, NACO, the Drug Controller General and the Ministry of Patents with the aim of developing a policy paper on the issue.

UNAIDS is planning to document best practices on HIV care and support in India. Under the aegis of International Alliance on HIV/AIDS. UNAIDS will build on these efforts.

UNAIDS has also advocated the formulation of legal and ethical guidelines approved by NACO for health care settings. UNAIDS, alongwith WHO, also supported a meeting held at the Asia Region level on Vaccine Development and Ethics.

Emerging Issues and Challenges

UNAIDS is at the core of a complex net of institutions. This strategic positioning being a strength, has also created challenging situations for the Programme's functioning. Thus, effective management of this network has been crucial in determining the strengths and weaknesses of the organisation. Functioning through a non-vertical structure and by developing mechanisms such as the Virtual Team has enabled the programme to integrate perspectives from different organisations.

UNAIDS has achieved a substantial degree of success in putting systems into place in several areas of intervention keeping the important goal of de-centralization in mind. It has due to its position in the global scenario, been successful in putting together resources and information in the form of global best practices. Being a part of the UN system puts UNAIDS at an advantage of taking several supporting stands, which it might not have been able to do otherwise.

Having come thus far into fighting the epidemic, UNAIDS has now to weigh carefully its future decisions keeping in perspective the current attitude of the Government, particularly because the main purpose of developing a collaborative framework is to ascertain that inputs are fed in appropriately into the National response. In this regard, some of the challenges that lie ahead for the organisation include the following:

Scaling up Interventions

Whereas a long term goal of the Organisation would be to support and strengthen the National Programme to facilitate an effective National response to the HIV epidemic, there are several challenges and risks in reaching the perceived objecting. Numbers in India and its diversity are serious factors which impact on the strategy and planning of HIV/AIDS interventions.

The challenge therefore lies in scaling up interventions at the same time, maintaining their quality to ascertain effective behaviour change. While many efforts have been made to fight the rising epidemic, there is still an enormous need for continued attention to program design and implementation throughout the country.

Strengthening Advocacy

Although, a major focus of the current program is on decentralization, the diverse nature of the epidemic across different states makes it difficult to maintain a uniform strategy. UNAIDS has a critical responsibility in strengthening linkages between states and TRGs so that the diverse needs can be met appropriately. There are plans to include the private sector more intensively in this area. Whether the corporate sector is willing to accept the HIV/AIDS issue as a development threat remains to be seen. Concerted advocacy will, therefore, have to be undertaken on this issue.

Strengthening a Co-ordinated Response

UNAIDS plays a major role in coordinating the response of the UN system to the epidemic. While the UN Agencies have responded well to the efforts and support of UNAIDS, the response of the national machinery to this joint effort will have to be reinforced further. For instance, an endeavour would have to be made to see how other ministries can merge HIV into their existing structures.

Multisectoral Response

Another major objective of UNAIDS is to strengthen a multisectoral, scaled up decentralised response to HIV/AIDS. This goal is again dependent on several factors. Many of the efforts such as the Virtual Team, and introduction of a more IT educated system are new and the response of the states and SACS will have to be studied carefully.

Would SACS be aggreable in accepting inputs from TRGs? Would they be in consonance with VT recommendations? Would they have the strength to use a proposed M&E framework and analyse the data? Would TRGs be able to suitably respond to the state needs? These are only some of the many issues which need to be carefully addressed.

In sum, although UNAIDS has made substantial efforts in meeting its objectives, in reality the HIV/AIDS raises social, ethical, moral and personal issues that are had to put forth us the public domain.

UNAIDS India will continue to endeavour towards fighting these challenges. It will work for strengthening a coordinated response, facilitating innovative efforts of its stakeholders and ascertaining more involvement of positive people in tackling the

HIV epidemic. It will work towards harnessing a common and evolving understanding of the epidemic in India within a larger framework of the development challenges which the country continues to face, so as to help maintain an effective National response.

References

1. *Source: A Strategic Response to the HIV Epidemic by the Government of India, the UN Agencies and its Development Partners in India*, UNAIDS, 1999.
2. *Source:* Strengthening State Responses to the Epidemic, 2nd HIV/AIDS Strategic Planning Retreat, Final Report.
3. Sen Biswajit, UNAIDS in India: Towards a Strategic Plan, July 2000.
4. UNAIDS Geneva. HIV and AIDS related stigmatization, discrimination and denial: forms, contexts and determinants - Research Studies from India and Uganda, June 2000.
5. Refer "Strategic Response to the HIV Epidemic "by the Govt. of India, the UN and Development partners in India.
6. NACO Report, 2000.
7. Report on the Global HIV/AIDS Epidemic, June 2000, UNAIDS.
8. For more information visit www.unaids.org
9. With inputs from Anne Vincent, Project Officer Health, UNICEF, India, Focal Point, Virtual Team
10. UNAIDS Report, 2000, Geneva.

Six

UNAIDS Best Practice Criteria: Projects Reviewed

I Effectiveness

Effectiveness is an activity's overall achievement in producing desired results and reaching overall objectives. Thus, to identify a project's effectiveness, one needs to know objectives and outcomes, as well as what changed during the time the activity was implemented and why the change took place. Whenever present, stated objectives differed widely, as did reported effectiveness measures (See Annexures). Some projects aimed simply to train healers and measured their effectiveness according to the number of healers trained and the information understood by healers. Others aimed to train traditional healers to reach fellow-healers, or the community served by healers, with AIDS information. Other projects aimed to alter the sexual practices of healers' clients or community members. Lastly, an aim of many projects was to strengthen collaboration between traditional healers and their biomedical counterparts. Measures of effectiveness in each of these cases comprised numbers of healers or community members trained by trained healers, behaviour change among healers' clients and/or community members, and collaboration indicators like referral between healers and biomedical health facilities or links built between healers and health structures.

All the eight projects compared in this study have described a substantial increased in knowledge among trained healers regarding symptoms of HIV disease, HIV transmission and prevention and whether or not AIDS was curable. One project in South Africa indicated an increase in positive attitudes about AIDS. Other measures of effectiveness included enumerating how much of the information trained healers passed on to fellow-healers or clients and community members.

In Botswana, healers trained in a two-week 'peer education' programme not only re-collected information they learned two years after training, but they professed to be training fellow-healers and community members as well. In Mozambique, South Africa, and Uganda, investigation showed that traditional healers were counseling clients in HIV/AIDS prevention and care. In Malawi, Uganda and the United Republic of Tanzania, trained healers were stated to be giving effective AIDS education, with the help of drama, song, dance and by developing their own training materials. In all except one of the eight projects studied here (the exception being Central African Republic, where investigators only measured change in knowledge), traditional healers were stated to be active condom promoters and distributors. Even after one-day training sessions, healers in Malawi stated having open discussions about condoms, and female traditional healers reported distributing condoms as often as male traditional healers.

II Ethical Soundness

Ethical soundness is ascertained in keeping with the principles of appropriate and acceptable social and professional conduct. Important concepts to be kept in mind regarding ethical soundness include: confidentiality, mutual respect, community and government participation, and informed consent. Ways of promoting ethical soundness adopted by most of the eight projects reviewed here included creating a climate of mutual respect between traditional healers and biomedical health practitioners, singing agreements or working closely with hospitals or the Ministry of Health, and ascertaining confidentiality of patients. Most projects were associated with the Ministry of Health, but only two of them reported that they informed traditional healers and their communities of the projects' results (i.e. provided feedback). The Malawi project specifically dealt with issues related to the negative or positive images reflected in awareness messages. Some projects also gave special attention to tailoring their messages to fit the understanding of traditional healers, or to strengthening aid in disadvantaged communities. Two issues of particular relevance to traditional medicine projects are:

(1) whether any patients experience harmful effects from traditional methods or treatments; and

(2) respect of the proprietary rights of traditional healers over their herbal preparations.

In the survey sent to project leaders to gather information for this report, none of the respondents indicated any harmful effects of herbal remedies and only one project discussed the measures in place to insure healers' rights over their treatments. Most of the projects reviewed here met the UNAIDS Best Practice criteria for ethical soundness. This criteria was not necessarily addressed as part of a systematic plan, but out of concern and respect for traditional healers, their clients and communities. A systematic plan to approach ethical soundness could include the following issues:

(a) Approval by scientific and ethical communities;
(b) Equal participation by males and females;
(c) Awareness of objectives and implications of project;
(d) Patient confidentiality;
(e) Safeguard of proprietary nights of traditional healers;
(f) Verifying any damage done by traditional healers; and
(g) Ensuring feedback from programme participants.

III Efficiency

Interest in efficiency has grown in off late with the realization of depletion of resources and their need to be used in the most cost-effective manner. The basic implication of efficiency is the ability to produce the desired results with least expenditure of energy, time, or resources. There are several economic evaluation techniques concerned with measuring cost-effectiveness, but they all involve knowing the costs involved in project implementation and concrete measures of effectiveness. Since most of the projects reviewed did not describe measures of efficiency, costs involved in various activities, or clear measures of effectiveness, it is difficult to form any opinion on this aspect. Efficiency, indicators in the various projects included:

(i) total cost of training each healer and each client or community member reached (see Annexure 3).
(ii) target number of traditional healers' clients and community members reached by healer initiatives (community AIDS education, drama, counselling).
(iii) target number of persons living with HIV/AIDS reached during home-care visits.

(iv) target number of fellow healers trained by trained traditional healers.
(v) existence of financial control
(vi) regularity of activity and financial reports.

In the three projects that reported the cost of training, the figures varied slightly. In Zambia, training costs were US$35, per day per traditional healer, in Botswana US$22, and in Uganda US$20. The figures available indicate that healers are able to attract large numbers of people to their community AIDS events, which results into very large numbers of people qualifying for education, once healers are trained. The Tanzania AIDS Working Group estimated that, in three years, some 27,000 community members were covered educational sessions, 4,300 persons living with HIV/AIDS in home visits and 450,000 people in drama groups. THETA Uganda estimates that it covers between 150,000 and 400,000 beneficiaries per year (thus between 450,000 and 1,200,000 in three years). In comparison, another AIDS educational strategy in Uganda - the AIDS education through Imams initiative-states that they have covered 100,000 homes in five years (UNAIDS, 1998a) - a similar level. The cost per beneficiary was only available for THETA Uganda, where it was estimated to be between US$0.24 and US$0.71 per year (see Annexure 4). One analysis in Botswana estimated that 30 per cent of persons living with HIV/AIDS would be admitted to a hospital during the course of their illness.

It was estimated that each user would average one re-admission, with each stay averaging 8.2 days and costing US$42 per day. Without home- or healer-based care, hospital treatment would cost US$241 per person living with HIV/AIDS (Cameron et al, 1994). Indicators that efficiency issues were being addressed included the presence of reporting and control of finances and administration. At THETA Uganda, accounts are audited annually and activity and financial reports are taken out quarterly. Financial administration is tightly controlled.

IV Sustainability

Sustainability is the ability of a programme to carry on with a certain degree of autonomy and to continue effective by over the medium-to-long term. For the projects reviewed here, sustainability was measured by finding out whether the information and skills passed on to healers were retained, and whether these skills were used over time. For instance, an assessment was made of whether healers continued to practice counselling, condom distribution, and community AIDS education, and whether they were still collaborating with biomedical health practitioners. The eight projects mainly tried to ascertain sustainability by building relations with health structures so that traditional healers could continue to receive support for their educational activities - including condoms for distribution - after completion of the intervention. None of the projects indicated paying healers' salaries, but they often reimbursed expenses such as transportation costs to reach training sites. Many projects assumed that even though project activities officially ended, healers had gained enough insight and skills to continue to use that information in their practices. This point has been reinforced by a number of different projects. Interviews conducted in Botswana Central African Republic and Zambia, years after the completion of training projects, revealed that healers recalled information imparted in training and that they were still using it through counselling and by educating clients and communities, as well as referring patients to hospitals and clinics.

The South African healers who were trained by fellow-healers felt confident to train a third generation of healers, but some of them preferred to be assisted by a project facilitator during training. Project design generally included information in their curricula, but often failed to identify the importance of incorporating into training the necessary skill-building sessions that would enable traditional healers to teach fellow-healers. In Uganda, healers who were trained during 1993-1994 continued to give education sessions in their communities and even started formal training of fellow-healers on their own initiative. Though THETA does not train the same healers it trained in 1993-1994, it is available to act as a guarantor for traditional healers' fund-raising, or to enable occasional workshops organized by healers.

Thus, sustainability is one of the most challenging issues facing HIV prevention efforts in general, and traditional medicine collaborative projects are no exception. One major difficulty is the definition and importance of sustainability given by different funders. This review points out that it has been extremely difficult for the majority of projects to remain active or to follow up with participating traditional healers over the long term, even though traditional healers remain active independently. A more systematic and standardized approach to sustainability is needed in order to design long-term projects and measure their impact over time.

Sustainability issues

Sustainability of results

(a) Are the results of the intervention permanent or temporary?
(b) Will new knowledge and activities (such as counselling and/or community education) continue even after training has ceased?

Funding

(a) Whether the project completely depends on external funding?
(b) Whether the project would continue if external funding were cut?
(c) Whether there are any income-generating activities within the projects?
(d) Whether there been any input of local aid, including volunteer labour or donations?

Capacity-building

(a) Whether there are any measures of capacity-building within the project's goals/ objectives?
(b) Whether traditional healers participated in design, implementation, or evaluation of project activities?

Local ownership

(a) What is the feeling among staff and community feel about the success or failure of the project?
(b) Is there a feeling of personal investment in the project by staff and community?

Links with local health or community systems

(a) Has the project built links with the hospital or clinics within the project area?

(b) Has the project made links with other community systems?
(c) How will these links be pursued over time?

V Relevance

It has been formally understood since the late 1970s that, for developing countries, it is imperative to involve traditional healers in primary health care (WHO, 1978). Since the early 1990s, the same applies for AIDS, especially in sub-Saharan Africa, where ministries of health cannot pay for adequate health care services. In addition, the large direct and indirect costs associated with AIDS in many countries make the need of cooperating with traditional healers all the more appealing. This it has been recognized that African healers are accessible, affordable, and culturally appropriate and acceptable, thereby fulfilling the major criteria for low-cost, effective health care service delivery in most sub-Saharan African settings. Therefore, the relevance of the overall approach of working with healers will be taken as assumed instead, it is the relevance of specific strategies used by particular projects that will be examined. Relevance signifies how closely a project is focused on the HIV/AIDS response in the context of the society in which it is implemented. Issues such as cultural and political factors are usually taken into account.

For the projects compared here, the emphasis was placed on how adequate the particular strategy of each project was to the HIV/AIDS situation and how project objectives were associated to the prevalence of HIV, needs assessments and the priorities of the National AIDS Programme. For instance, countries with a mature epidemic should combine prevention with counselling and care, as was done in the project in the United Republic of Tanzania. In the projects reviewed in Annexure 3, objectives were defined following baseline research with traditional healers, implemented either through surveys or focus group discussions. In only some projects was it mentioned that needs were examined according to the larger political context - specifically with reference to the AIDS epidemiology - or the surrounding community needs. However, in most of the countries in this review, the prevalence of HIV was already high when the projects were begun.

The difference in political will to work with traditional healers among countries can play a strong part in the overall accomplishment of this type of collaborative project, but this was seldom mentioned in project literature. THETA Uganda was the only project that carried out needs assessment in communities surrounding the traditional healers. Three projects indicated that their objectives were directly based on National AIDS Programme priorities. The Malawi project noted that its objectives changed alongwith the AIDS situation. In the Central African Republic, it was observed that the content of the training curriculum was relevant to all types of healers trained, as the degree of knowledge and attitude change was not related to traditional healers' characteristics.

Thus, measures of relevance varied widely in the different contexts of the projects reviewed. Where the relevance of involving traditional healers in HIV/AIDS control efforts is no longer important, it is necessary that the objectives and strategies used by each project be according to the given context. This will have a considerable impact on effectiveness. Issues to consider regarding the project relevance are listed below:

Relevance issues

Needs assessment

(a) Whether the project hold a needs assessment study before developing objectives?

HIV/AIDS Context

(a) Whether the project taken into account the local HIV prevalence, incidence and other AIDS interventions?

Relevance to National AIDS Programme priorities

(a) Whether the project considered the priorities of the National AIDS Programme?

Political context

(a) Whether the project considered the political, social and cultural context surrounding traditional medicine, AIDS and other STD issues?

Consideration Applicable to Traditional Medicine and Biomedicine Collaborative Projects

Factors to be considered before selecting 'genuine' of 'authentic' healers

Due to the absence of regulatory bodies for traditional healers in most countries, selection of 'genuine' or 'authentic' healers can be a challenge for most new projects. In this regard, the eight projects under study mainly consulted community leaders, traditional healer associations and the ministries incharge of traditional healer activities for approval and for recommendations of genuine or authentic healers. Many project leaders remarked on the extensive time needed to select genuine traditional healers who were truly interested in collaboration. In Senegal, basis for selection were initially founded on healers' reputations. The selection was improved by the use of children, considered innocent and unbiased. They were questioned as to which healer in their community they would refer someone with an ailment. In South Africa, the project first reached five traditional healers' associations to choose healers for training. However, in the second round of training, it was noticed that the trained healers were much more effective at selecting genuine healers than the traditional healers' associations were. Other initiatives also found that it was better to avoid traditional healers' associations, as the internal politics of these associations can sometimes hinder the selection, training, or other project objectives. Such was the case in Uganda, where the criteria for traditional healers' selection used by THETA are the following:

(a) being recognized as healers by the community and local authorities;
(b) having regular patient attendance;
(c) having a clinic or shrine to receive and treat patients; and
(d) knowing how to prepare herbal remedies.

Considering the following issues can be useful in selecting healers to participate in collaborative projects.

Community recommendations; Traditional healers' associations recommendations; Ministry recommendations; Do the traditional healers selected have regular patient attendance? Do the traditional healers use Herbal preparations; Does the project take time to select genuine traditional healers.

Establishing trust with traditional healers

Discussion, interviews and listening to traditional healers' needs were the most common ways of building trust with traditional healers, and it was accepted that doing this gradually without rushing the traditional healers, was necessary. In Uganda, clear recognition of healers' rights to their treatment secrets was stressed in order to help gain trust in setting up the initial collaborative clinical research on herbal treatments for opportunistic infections. In both the United Republic of Tanzania and Uganda, a series of workshops were organized after initial contacts to share ideas between representatives of the two health care systems. Other methods used repeated visits to healers' homes/clinics or focus group discussions as a way of establishing trust. Considering the following issues can be useful in building trust among traditional healers:

Taking time to build strong relationships; Treating traditional healer participants with respect; Recognizing traditional healers' proprietary right to their treatments.

Lessons Learned

Training methods

The Government of South Africa recently hired a traditional healer to regularly train fellow-healers. With her many years of experience, this traditional healer suggested that traditional healers need a participatory approach to training, and need to be shown the utmost respect. She advised, "Let them burn their incense in training", meaning that if the project respects the traditional healers' customs, the training will be successful. In addition, she emphasized the importance of using fellow-healers to train others, as healers are more receptive to hearing new things from their peers. She cautions against talking about traditional healers' associations in training as the politics will distract healers from the training session (Manci, 1999, personal communication). Other project leaders agreed with Manci about the issue of respect and some specifically emphasized the importance of respecting healers as professional health care providers.

With regard to content of training, most initiatives have had little difficulty with issues around AIDS symptoms, HIV transmission and prevention, condom use, condom promotion and distribution. The areas that provided the biggest obstacles were home care, death and dying, mother-to-child HIV transmission and, in the Central African Republic, condom use, which the authors linked to a high desire to have children.

Collaboration

Healers in Uganda and the United Republic of Tanzania have been given access to hospitals, which has motivated them greatly. One project leader in the United Republic of Tanzania suggested establishing a cooperative relationship with a hospital or clinic to facilitate collaboration (Scheinman, personal communication). THETA Uganda leaders noted as well that developing a lasting collaboration between the two health systems involves much effort on both sides of the collaborative relationship. Collaborative project designs cannot emphasize only the efforts required by healers and assume that the biomedical health workers will follow without as much time and energy input. In Malawi, similar lessons were noted, and authors suggested that more collaborative referral networks need to be encouraged between traditional healers and the formal health sector (Porter, 1996). It may be that what is needed is simply a change of attitude within the biomedical health structures and among personnel. The key is a true dialogue (Webb, 1997).

Finally, THETA has suggested that the type of collaboration they have created in Uganda could be extended nationwide if emphasis were placed on building strong links at the community level with local leaders, health authorities, government and non-governmental key players. These links ensure sustainability, reduce programme costs and increase healer recognition in their own communities.

Project Design and Implementation

One of the most important lessons learned is not only that collaboration is possible, but that it has yielded valuable public health benefits. As longer-term projects have revealed, it is often not until after training that trained heaters devise innovative initiatives for HIV prevention. For example, in Mozambique, it was noted that some trained traditional healers shared the information they gained from one workshop with other healers in their traditional healers' association. This may be evidence that the training was valued enough that some healers expanded the training without asking for resources. It is therefore critical to plan and secure funding for long-term monitoring, evaluation and follow-up of collaborative Projects.

Given the changing epidemic and the dynamic relationship between the two health sectors, this issue becomes even more crucial if we are to take advantage of, and learn from, this exploratory field.

Conclusion

The review of the various projects has suggested that a systematic evaluation of collaborative projects is urgently needed, especially to find out determinants of success and/or failure. Since many of the projects are still in an experimental stage, the information collected could be used to modify existing efforts and help develop new ones. Various variables need to be assessed for this and it is only with systematic and repeated evaluations, using a variety of technologies, that we can hope to answer some of the major questions we are faced with. There is lack of rigorous, long-term measures of effectiveness and sustainability. Of particular interest is the question of cost-effectiveness. None of the projects reviewed here officially reported on the efficiency of training with respect to cost-effectiveness. Unfortunately, without cost-effectiveness data the funding agencies easily deny the need of such projects. Research, not just of the methods that traditional healers use and the impact of training projects, but also into the link between the traditional and biomedical health care systems, is important so as to answer questions about collaboration between the two systems. How each health systems influences the other, and how the relationship could be mutually beneficial, need to be known in order to build a sustainable relationship between the two sectors. With greater focus on home care since the advent of AIDS, it is possible that traditional healers may act as a crucial link in the continuum of care from hospital to home.

Research into the healer approach to care is another neglected sphere of research that shows great promise. An in-depth analysis of the counselling given by traditional healers, and how they biomedical concepts into their traditional belief system and methods of practice, merge needs to be examined research as it is important while understanding the impact traditional healers could have in both care and prevention of STDs and HIV/AIDS. In the ongoing struggle to give comprehensive health care to a diverse population, research into the role of traditional healers could result in the development of innovative new strategies. For instance, since the mid-1990s, traditional healers have played an increasingly important role in the promotion of condoms in some countries in Africa. It is thus possible for them to play a part in providing greater access to other health care choices such as family planning. This area has been looked at in some countries for primary health care, but has not spread to other areas of health or examined on a large scale. The goal of maximizing availability of drugs in indigent countries makes research on herbal medicine crucial today. The question regarding standardization and regulation of traditional medicine training and traditional healers' practice has been considered with respect to creating national policies.

Agreement has not yet been reached, but the issues are complex as acceptance often depends on organisation of traditional healers. There is fear that regulation and standardization of traditional healers' practices will resulting loss of diversity within these practices. However, many traditional healers are still keen on recognition by the biomedical structure and welcome official policy changes to this effect. Collaborative projects have much to gain from each other. A modified system of communication among traditional healers, as well as among countries, would be useful. Regular meetings and networking would advantage not only the projects concerned but also their beneficiaries.

ANNEXURE 1
REVIEW OF EXAMPLES OF COLLABORATION ACCORDING TO UNAIDS BEST PRACTICE CRITERIA

*Project**	*Effectiveness*	*Ethical soundness*	*Efficiency*	*Sustainability*	*Relevance of approach*
Dingaka AIDS Awareness, **Botswana** 1991-1993	- Trained traditional healers passed on information to clients and fellow-traditional healers - 80% of traditional healers recommend condoms to patients - 31/32 refer patients - Nurses refer to traditional healers	- Programme worked with Ministry of Health	- Estimated cost US$22 per traditional healer trained per day - Traditional healers trained, on average, 45 other traditional healers per district	- Not sustainable as a project, but healers have continued to use the information they gained.	- Objectives clearly stated, and relevant to the AIDS situation, but TOT and collaboration aspects of the project ambitious for time and resources allocated.
Action to Define, Broaden, and Strengthen the Role of Traditional Practitioners (ADERT) **Central African Republic** 1994	- Significant improvement in traditional healers' knowledge on STD risk, condom use, and HIV transmission after training - 76% of traditional healers with STD cases report integrating partner referral into their STD care treatment.	- Programme worked with Ministry of Health - Specific attention to appropriateness of training topics and methods for traditional healers	- 103 traditional healers trained in 4 locations over 2 months - No cost-effectiveness measures	- No measures taken to ensure sustainability; activities ceased when funding stopped. - One healer interviewed in 1999 said he was eager to be involved in another project and he was still using the information gained.	- Objectives clearly stated and relevant to needs assessed through baseline focus group discussion and working group of traditional healers and Ministry of Health staff. - Magnitude of knowledge and attitude change was no related to traditional healers' characteristics, indicating that impact of training was uniform among practitioners. The implies that specific types of practitioners do not need targeting, and training content was relevant to all traditional healers in that setting and context.

*Project**	*Effectiveness*	*Ethical soundness*	*Efficiency*	*Sustainability*	*Relevance of approach*
Training on AIDS for traditional healers **Malawi** 1992	- Increase in traditional healers' knowledge - 64% conducted AIDS education events - 89% distributed condoms - No evaluation of collaboration.	- Collaboration with Malawi NACP - The purpose of the study was clearly explained to each traditional healer - Specific attention to positive images in educational messages	- In 6 months, 3000 community members reached in AIDS education	- Most healers within walking distance of training. - Traditional healers encouraged to acquire condoms from health centre.	- Goals and objectives clearly stated and relevant to needs assessed through baseline survey. - Project changed significantly in response to changes in AIDS situation. - Strategy did not include specific emphasis on biomedical health sector.
Ministry of Health/traditional healers' association collaboration **Mozambique** 1991-1994	- 85% traditional healers able to describe HIV symptoms - 85% knew AIDS transmitted by sex - 81% traditional healers promoting condom use - traditional healers advise clients to avoid having many sex partners	- Programme started by Ministry of Health	- 47 traditional healers trained - No information on cost-effectiveness	- At least one follow-up workshop for traditional healers organized by the Provincial Health Dept. within 10 months of the initial workshop. - Traditional healers reported distributing condoms and cooperating in other area with health department	- Objectives clearly stated and based on preliminary ethnomedical research, taking into consideration the national and local STD/AIDS programme priorities, as well as the political situation.

*Project**	*Effectiveness*	*Ethical soundness*	*Efficiency*	*Sustainability*	*Relevance of approach*
Training of trainers **South Africa** 1992	- Traditional healers training other traditional healers, counselling clients, promoting condoms. - Increased positive attitudes	- Collaboration with traditional healers' associations	- 1510 traditional healers trained, all but 28 by fellow-traditional healers in almost 1 year	- Second-generation traditional healers were prepared to train third-generation healers with minimal assistance	- Objectives clearly stated and based on feasibility of engaging traditional healers in the fight against AIDS
Traditional and Modern Health Practitioners Together against AIDS (THETA) **Uganda** 1992	- 200 traditional healers trained in 7 districts since 1993 - Traditional healers gained knowledge in HIV/AIDS and STD transmission, prevention and care - Traditional healers gained counselling, teaching, leadership and record-keeping skills. - Trained traditional healers providing regular community AIDS education - Traditional healers distributing condoms - Traditional healers make increased referrals to biomedical health providers - THETA produces a newsletter, initiated a speakers' bureau, contains a library on traditional medicine and AIDS, and produced 2 videos - Conducted a study on the effectiveness of herbal treatment for opportunistic infections.	- Research results are fed back to healers and community - Patient confidentiality is emphasized in training programmes - Agreement signed with Ministry of Health - Traditional healers have worked within the hospital for herbal study - Patients sign informed consent form - Mutual respect is emphasized from the beginning	- Admin. tightly controlled and reports produced quarterly - Costs per traditional healer client range between US$ 0.24 and US$ 0.71 - US$ 21/day per traditional healer trained - Estimated total number of beneficiaries range from 150,000 to 400,000 per year*	- Healers don't receive salaries - Strong links are built with community leaders in each district (i.e. local council, secretaries for women, etc.) for supporting continuing healer activities - Traditional healers involved in the training have formed their own associations that undertake various activities, including community AIDS education and drama, training of fellow-healers, and 'persons living with HIV/AIDS' support groups - THETA trained traditional healers involved in national policy bodies (National Drug Authority)	- Objectives clearly stated and based on baseline traditional healers' surveys and community baseline assessments - Objectives and implementation follow the National AIDS Programme strategy - Implementation of district activities is area-specific and based on feasibility assessments carried out in several possible sites before each new district is chosen

Project*	Effectiveness	Ethical soundness	Efficiency	Sustainability	Relevance of approach
Tanga AIDS Working Group, (TAWG) **United Republic of Tanzania** 1990	- 120 traditional healers trained since 1994 - Drama group reached 55,000 people in 4 months - 1997 survey showed traditional healers had increased awareness of HIV/AIDS - Clients who were counselled reduced risky behaviour	- Mutual respect is a main TAWG principle - Counselled patients are given code numbers and confidentiality is assured - Ministry of Health authorised research; offices within hospital - Research results fed back to healers and NGO	- Traditional treatments are free for patients - In 3 years: 27000 community members reached in education sessions - 237 persons living with HIV/AIDS reached in 4,300 home-care visits	- As permanent members of the community, traditional healers will continue to practise their new research and counselling skills even if the NGO is not present - Healers don't receive salaries - NGO office is in the hospital; links between hospital and NGO are strong - 17 supervisors from the health facilities were trained to monitor and support traditional healers.	- Objectives clearly stated and based on 7 years of experience working with traditional healers. - Linking prevention and care provides a culturally relevant approach for the Tanga region.
AIDS research, training and follow-up **Zambia** 1994-1996	- 250 traditional healers promoting and selling condoms - Traditional healers counselling on HIV and STD prevention, HIV testing and caring for persons living with HIV/AIDS at home	- Ministry of Health agreement - Project planned for feedback of results to province, district and local levels	- US$35/day per traditional healers trained	- Links built between traditional healers and local biomedical health practitioner and health facility	- Objectives clearly stated and based on preliminary assessments and national AIDS programme priorities.

For ongoing project, only starting date given.

*Calculations are explained in Table 4.

ANNEXURE 2
SPECIFIC CRITERIA/APPROACH FOR COLLABORATION

Country	*Criteria for selecting 'genuine' or 'authentic' healers*	*Approach used to build trust*	*Lessons learned*
Botswana	- Leaders from different traditional healers' associations in 6 districts selected 12 traditional healers for training	- Discussions and seminars with traditional healers	- Condom promotion easily integrated into traditional healers' practice - Home care difficult to integrate into traditional healers' practice - Follow-up necessary to sustain the intervention - Traditional healers see doctors as their counterparts - The legal status of traditional healers should be dealt with in order to improve organisation of traditional healers and ultimately improve cooperation between health sectors - Biomedical health practitioners should be trained to acknowledge that patients share traditional and modern beliefs and values
Central African Republic	- The most influential traditional healers were selected by village leaders from a census list of traditional healers	- Central African Republic physician employed persistence, rapport building, and mobilizing skills to slowly gain trust. - Traditional healers slowly found that collaborating with Ministry of Health would legitimize them in the eyes of the government.	- Attitudes towards condom use did not change. Investigators linked this information to a high desire to have children. - Authors found that careful design of curriculum adapted for training of traditional healers is useful for traditional healers' increase in knowledge; a one-time training cannot achieve a significant level of change in traditional healers' practice. Rather a repetitive model would be most effective for promoting cognitive, attitudinal and behavioural change.

Country	Criteria for selecting 'genuine' or 'authentic' healers	Approach used to build trust	Lessons learned
Malawi	- Older healers were reported to have more credibility with village leaders - Community leaders were consulted to gain approval and to recommended the most respected and most active traditional healers in their areas	- Focus group discussions were held with groups of traditional healers to build relationships between healers, Ministry of Health and project.	- Traditional healers were open to condom promotion - Need for greater collaboration between health centre staff and traditional healers to maintain community-based education and condom distribution
Mozambique	- Traditional healers' association assisted in selection of traditional healer, seeking to provide balance by gender, age and district.	- In-depth interviews and focus group discussions over 9-month period before training.	- Much public health knowledge and practice is already found in beliefs and practices of traditional healers. Difficult to interview patients of traditional healers due to stigma of STDs. The use of indigenous disease name proved a great facilitator of communication as it was taken as a sign of respect.
Senegal	- Selection based on healers' reputation, and preschool children 4-6 years old were asked to identify traditional healers known for specific conditions	- Consent of local authorities - Series of contacts that lasted from several months to years - Healers provided names and addresses of other healers	- PROMETRA considers its work to be cultural research, medical practice, and views itself as an integral partner in dissemination of scientific information to a large community.
AIDS Foundation, **South Africa**	- Traditional healers themselves selected traditional healers to be trained	- Traditional healers approached the AIDS Foundation of South Africa for training	- Traditional healers identified the need for rural AIDS hospices and trained home-care personnel - More work needs to be done to eliminate the tenuous and strained aspect of the relationship between traditional healers and biomedical practitioners.

Country	*Criteria for selecting 'genuine' or 'authentic' healers*	*Approach used to build trust*	*Lessons learned*
Training of Trainers, **South Africa**	- 5 national traditional healers' associations selected traditional healers for first workshop based on gender and geographical balance. - Trained traditional healers selected healers for future workshops.	- In-depth interviews and focus group discussions over 1-year period.	- Misconceptions about AIDS are easily dispelled - Second-generation traditional healers were as well, if not better, trained than first-generation healers due to better selection of trainees by traditional healers - Training on death and dying was not liked by traditional healers. - It was advised to discontinue work with traditional healers' organisations to avoid political conflicts - Traditional healers wanted explicit condom demonstration - As traditional healers had access to intimate details of patients' physical emotional and spiritual lives, the experienced few problems influencing behaviour in sex and sexuality
Uganda	THETA selection criteria: - Being recognized as healers by their community and local authorities - Having regular patient attendance - Having a clinic or shrine to receive and treat patients - Knowing how to prepare herbal remedies - Questionnaire answered by each healer	- Emphasis on healers' right to ownership of their treatments. - Initial contact through the Culture Officer of the Ministry of Gender and Community Development as well as through a TASO doctor and personal visit to traditional healer's clinic	- Research with traditional healers requires mutual respect and collaboration with biomedical health practitioner - Collaborative work requires time to build trust and continuous follow-up to monitor and evaluate a changing epidemic, and a dynamic relationship between the 2 health sectors - Traditional healers can come up with innovative ideas for AIDS prevention long after training is completed. - This type of collaboration can extend nationwide if strong links are built at the community level with local leaders, government and nongovernmental key players and health authorities.

Country	Criteria for selecting 'genuine' or 'authentic' healers	Approach used to build trust	Lessons learned
United Republic of Tanzania	- Two types of participatory approaches were used to identify key traditional healers and health personnel to participate in the training workshops.	- Meetings were arranged between expatriate physical and traditional healers. Healers enjoyed being taken seriously and being treated like fellow professionals. Initial dialogues evolved into a series of workshops on patient care, treatment, education and cooperation between biomedical and traditional health practitioners.	- Traditional healers should be respected as health professionals - Give traditional healers access to hospitals, clinics, and patients - Involve them in home care and training - Healers care about their patients and want to learn more - Traditional healers are keen students. - Traditional healers love learning about research - Traditional healers enjoy mutual referral between them and hospital/clinics - Develop a cooperative and collaborative relationship between traditional healers and hospital/clinic
Zambia	- Traditional leaders assisted health centre staff in selection process. - Professional reputation within the community, willingness and ability to learn and communication skills.	- Training was highly participatory - Health workers facilitating workshops underwent training in participatory methods - Effort was made to find terms that are more familiar to traditional healers' understanding of health and disease rather than using biomedical terminology	- Traditional healers came up with symbolic alternatives to high risk practices - After culturally appropriate exposure to explanations of public health, traditional healers can modify ritual practices

ANNEXURE 3
Efficiency calculations for THETA Uganda

*Population in the districts targeted by THETA (1991)**	*Rural*	*Urban*	*Total*
Mbarara	884,156	46,616	930,772
Mukono	725,869	98,735	824,604
Kamuli	473,200	8,262	481,462
Soroti	384,116	46,274	430,390
Hoima	193,300	4,616	197,916
Kiboga	136,330	5,277	141,607
Total	*2,796,971*	*209,780*	*3,006,751*
Total Ugandan population 1991*			16,671,705
Estimated total Ugandan population 1998			22,000,000
Estimated population growth 1991-1998			*32%*
Estimated 1998 population of the 6 districts targeted by THETA	*3,690,886*	*276,826*	*3,967,712*
Traditional healer population estimates			
No. of traditional healers in the 6 districts targeted by THETA**			1,407
No. of traditional healers trained by THETA in all 6 districts (40 per district)			240
Percentage of traditional healers trained by THETA in all 6 districts			*17%*
Estimated beneficiaries			
Total estimated 1998 pop. of the 6 districts targeted by THETA	3,690,886	276,826	3,967,712
Estimated % population using THs Low estimate***	29%	20%	
Estimated number of people based on Low estimate***	1,070,357	55,365	1,125,722
Estimated % population using THs High estimate***	85%	75%	
Estimated number of people based on High estimate***	3,137,253	207,619	3,344,873
Estimated 1998 client population of THETA trained THs (17% of traditional healers trained by THETA)			
Based on low estimate of pop. using THs	182,577	9,444	912,021
Based on high estimate of pop. using THs	535,139	35,415	570,554

Estimated costs per beneficiary:

Training programme costs per year (1998 figure)	US$	128,722.00
Cost per trained traditional healer per year of training (240 -traditional healers)	US$	536.34
Cost per trained traditional healer per day of training (26 days/year)	US$	20.63
Cost per trained traditional healer per year of practice post-training		
assuming 5 years of practice post training	US$	107.27
assuming 10 years of practice post training	US$	53.63
Cost per traditional healer client, based on		
low estimate of pop. using THs- based on	US$	0.71
high estimate of pop. using THs	US$	0.24

* Based on the 1991 National Population and Housing Census.

** Based on figures submitted by community at country level for "individuals known to treat people spiritually or with herbs".

*** Based on references: Scheinman, 1997 (personal communication); Dupree et al, 1992; Barton & Wamai, 1994.

Seven

Prevention Strategies for HIV

Importance of Costing Analysis

The worldwide implementation of HIV prevention work has been on for more than a decade. In spite of this there is absence of any costing and cost analysis specific to this field. There is even less done regarding assessing the relative cost-effectiveness of different prevention strategies. Cost analysis is a tool that helps in providing useful insight into the functioning of projects, as well as being a key component of cost-effectiveness analysis. Within HIV prevention, cost analysis enable managers at project level decide upon the best way to deliver a particular strategy. Cost analysis will help managers in a number of ways, which include:

(a) giving an overview of the total amount of funds that are needed to begin or continue a project;
(b) examining the use of different inputs (such as staff or equipment) within a project, and assisting in discussions about the relative efficiency and equity of projects;
(c) guiding discussions about the best mix and volume of preventive strategies and the best way to allocate resources—for instance, whether more resources should be allocated to Sexually Transmitted Diseases (STD) services relative to media education;
(d) giving an estimate of the extent of resources required for enhancing or replicating interventions.

Cost and cost-effectiveness analyses help in giving basic evidence for on-going policy questions and debates. Cost analyses have always been connected with issues of efficiency, cost-recovery and sustainability of programmes. However, cost analysis can also play a crucial part in assessing issues of equity and targeting, which have recently come to the forefront of the policy debate.

With the current research and development of new HIV prevention strategies, the question of their adequacy is importantly associated with issues of cost, efficiency and priorities for resource allocation. Cost and cost-effectiveness analyses are even more relevant in this context.

Cost data from on-going HIV prevention activities initiate a more informed national and international debate. Prevention activities may be extremely diverse both within and between countries. Therefore, it is crucial that, although costing approaches will depend on the object of the specific exercise and on local circumstances, there is consistency in the costing methods used. In this way, work undertaken in one field can have maximum relevance to managers in other context.

The principles of these Costing Guidelines are obtained from Cost Analysis in Primary Health Care - a training manual for programme managers (hereafter referred to as the 'PHC Manual').[1] The manual was produced for programme managers to demonstrate how cost analysis might be used to answer basic questions about the efficiency, equity and sustainability of the health activities for which they were answerable. It was hoped that the use of cost analyses would help in making decisions about the optimal use of resources within the health sector and within individual programmes. The PHC Manual is one of a number of relevant costing manuals produced over recent years. Much of the guidance it provides is directly related to managers of AIDS programmes who want cost analysis to help in their own decision-making. Manual is reading for users.

As in the PHC Manual, these Guidelines cost projects from the perspective of service providers and not from a social perspective. This should be borne in mind when interpreting the findings of the costing studies. The relevance and clarity of the Guidelines have been tested by costing a sample of prevention projects in several countries. This experience has been fed into the revision of the Guidelines.

Aim of the Guidelines and Audience

The specific aim of these Guidelines is to encourage and enable managers of HIV prevention projects and programmes to conduct cost analysis. These Guidelines relate the costing methodology presented in the PHC Manual and adapted to HIV prevention activities. These Guidelines can be used to assess projects/programmes at national, regional, district and community levels. We do not assume any prior experience or training in economics for users of these Guidelines. Detailed exercises to practise concepts of cost analysis are found at the back of the PHC Manual.

Structure of the Guidelines

The Guidelines begin by introducing and describing different strategies for HIV prevention. Chapter 2 provides an introduction to the basic economic concepts of cost analysis, upon which these Guidelines are based. Chapter 3 takes the reader through a step-by-step guide to planning and undertaking a cost analysis, including how to collect data. Annex 1 provides the background worksheets for individuals wanting to undertake a cost analysis. Finally the Guidelines end with a section on relevant literature in the area of cost and cost-effectiveness of HIV prevention strategies. A Microsoft Excel version of the spreadsheet is available on the UNAIDS website (www.unaids.org/publications) or the CD-ROM: Economics in HIV/AIDS planning: getting priorities right, UNAIDS (June 2000).

So as to conduct a cost analysis of a project or programme, it is important to know how a project functions. This chapter provides an insight into different HIV prevention strategies and brings to light factors that are important to the collection of the cost data.

Established Prevention Strategies

Following are nine established AIDS strategies. They may be used individually or jointly. The Section further discusses the description of potential projects, and key variables that are likely to affect the costs of each strategy.

(i) Screening blood for HIV infection;
(ii) Use of the mass media;
(iii) AIDS education in schools;
(iv) Social marketing of condoms;
(v) Treatment of sexually transmitted diseases;

(vi) Commercial sex worker peer education;
(vii) Voluntary counselling and testing;
(viii) Prevention activities among injecting drug users, and
(ix) Prevention of mother-to-child/vertical transmission.

Screening Blood for HIV Infection

The object of HIV blood screening strategy is to reduce the estimated 5-10 per cent of HIV infections in developing countries that are transmitted through infected blood transfusions. This can be achieved almost completely through the testing of all blood donations for HIV antibodies before transfusion, and the rejecting of donations that test HIV-positive. HIV blood screening can only be conducted as an integral part of a more comprehensive blood transfusion service (BTS) but, in this study consideration of the strategy is restricted to the HIV blood-screening component. The methodology presented could be extended to cover the other possible components. The main activities undertaken by a BTS are:

(a) donor recruitment and selection;
(b) collection of blood;
(c) a variety of blood screening tests;
(d) blood processing, storage and distribution;
(e) final transfusion of the blood; and
(f) support activities such as management and administration and staff training.

A broader HIV blood safety strategy could include more activities, such as more rational use of blood transfusion by the health service and prevention of conditions that usually need blood transfusion as part of their treatment. Screening blood for HIV stands out on a member of counts from the other strategies that are discussed ahead.

Firstly, there is general consensus on the degree of the strategy's effectiveness. Consensus that more than 95 per cent of HIV-negative patients transfused with HIV-infected blood will be affected facilitates calculation of the number of cases of HIV infection preventable by HIV blood screening. Calculations are, however, based on the reliability of the blood tests, and the chances of transfusing infected blood. The number of units of blood testing false positive will depend on the specificity of the test as well as the presence of HIV in the donated blood.

Secondly, the accountability for HIV infection contracted through infected blood products lies almost completely with health services. Preventive action therefore also lies with them (in contrast to other strategies that emphasize on prevention through individual responsibility and altered behaviour). This can lead to a medical and political necessity to implement the strategy, irrespective of whether its cost-effectiveness is relative to alternative HIV prevention strategies. It can also make it the least politically sensitive HIV prevention strategy to put into practice.

Irrespective of the prevalence level of HIV, only a small percentage of the population, namely blood transfusion recipients, will benefit directly from the strategy. This leads to dispute over the priority to be given to HIV blood screening. On the one hand, it is recommended that only at certain levels of HIV prevalence will HIV blood screening be a cost-effective strategy to pursue. On the other hand, it is suggested that no unscreened blood should be transfused, except in life-saving situations. More information on the costs and effectiveness of implementing HIV screening strategies may reduce the degree of controversy. Political and ethical considerations ensure that no country would be able, or inclined, to have a policy of transfusing, untested blood due to want of resources necessary for HIV screening and their better use elsewhere.

In presenting the costs of the HIV blood screening strategy, other indirect gains of the strategy should also be pointed out. These may include reduced transmission of other blood-acquired infections such as hepatitis B and syphilis (which results from the more comprehensive screening procedures established in conjunction with the HIV screening strategy), and enhanced reach to blood transfusions. A detailed manual on costing blood transfusion services is available from WHO.

Potential projects: Examples of ways of Implementation

The nature of BTS projects can be very variable and onc of the early jobs of the costing exercise will be to describe the particular one to be costed. BTS may be integrated with other health services, often as part of hospital services, or may be run independently from other health services in a vertical fashion. Costing is likely to be simple in the latter case, where the services are more easily demarcated, than when they are integrated with other activities.

The strategic responses of countries to the risk of HIV transmission through blood will also be variable and context-specific. The costs of adding HIV screening procedures to an established BTS may be quite less. For some countries, however, to provide HIV-screened blood may involve major reorganisation of the BTS. Some examples of the ways in which HIV blood screening strategies may be implemented:

(i) Countries without formal blood transfusion services may collect and transfuse blood as and when required. In this case, the HIV blood screening strategy is likely to be decentralized and involve one-test screening procedures at peripheral locations.

(ii) Countries may organize decentralised use of test kits as in (i), but supplement this with more centralised arrangements for additional testing of the positive tests.

(iii) Regional blood banks may be set up with their own laboratory blood-testing facilities or with samples being sent to a more central facility for HIV testing. At this organisational level and above, techniques like pooling blood for testing may be used to decrease costs. Decentralized use of one-test kits may still be suitable in peripheral services.

(iv) The national BTS may be centralized with all blood collected and tested centrally and HIV-screened blood distributed from the centre. Decentralized use of one-test kits may still be suitable in case of peripheral services.

These are only a few instances of an array of possible options for responding to the risk of HIV transmission through infected blood. Clearly, the nature of the services will greatly influence their costs, and these will vary from one model to another. In undertaking costing and cost-effectiveness analyses of BTS, it is important to recognize that different country analyses will rarely be dealing with directly comparable systems.

Variables which Affect Costs

Other than the cost implications of organisational and structural differences between different BTS outlined in above, there are other factors that differ between projects that affect absolute costs and relative cost-effectiveness. Some of these are highlighted as follows:

(a) *HIV prevalence in the recipient and donor population:* Firstly, in case of recipients: there is no HIV infection which can be averted if a clean unit of blood is transfused to a patient if he is already HIV-positive. Secondly in case of the donors: if the prevalence of HIV in donated blood is 20 per cent, then the amount of blood discarded would be likely to be twice as much as when the prevalence is only 10 per cent. This will have an impact on the costs of replacing blood and the cost per HIV infection averted.

(b) *Donor recruitment policies:* HIV-infected donations will be much less if steps are taken to exclude donors at high risk of HIV infection and to recruit only low-risk voluntary donors. For example, in Zambia, schoolchildren are the principal population from whom blood is collected. This requires widespread travel by mobile blood collection teams. The cost of transport is high, which is offset by the much-reduced need to discard blood.

(c) *Whether blood samples or the patients are the focus of HIV testing:* Where patients are the focus, the method in which HIV-positive donors are counselled will have resource implications. Sometimes positive tests may lead to counselling of infected patients and tracing of their sexual contacts; sometimes to counselling of the patient only; and sometimes just the discarding of the donation is enough and no personal contact is required with the patient.

(d) *Economies of scale at different organisational levels:* For instance, where blood is collected, tested and transfused on demand at the local level, costs for recruitment, collection, storage and transport will be relatively less than they are in more structured services. The amount of blood collected at the local level will determine whether or not pooled or bulk testing of blood can be carried out. At the national level, the size of the BTS will determine the scale of operations and influence unit costs.

(e) *The type of HIV tests being used:* Although the costs of HIV tests have been declining in recent years, the rapid serological tests is still more expensive (per unit tested) than testing a large batch using an ELISA test. However, depending on the volume and how often the blood is collected, the use of an ELISA reader may or may not be economical. The number of additional tests used as controls also depends on the number of units being tested at once. Rapid tests use essentially one control per test, whereas an ELISA test will use, at most, one for every six tests. This will affect the total costs of testing.

(f) *The reliability of the HIV tests used:* Wrong tests will lead to the wastage of good blood and the transfusion of infected blood. However, most tests now have high levels of sensitivity and specificity.

(g) *Whether laboratory costs are exclusively on HIV blood testing* or are shared with other laboratory services.

(h) *The order in which different tests are conducted* (e.g. HIV, hepatitis, syphilis and blood grouping) will affect the costs when the blood is discarded and not tested further if it tests positive for any one test. The most cost-effective order will be a factor of the relative costs of the tests and the prevalence of each condition in the donor population, which will in turn effect the probability of each test leading to discarding of the blood. However, not all services operate in this fashion, and sometimes all tests are carried out before any blood is discarded.

(i) *The skill mix of staff implementing the strategy:* The skill mix of the staff may also effect the degree to which choices are made between ELISA and rapid tests.

Use of the Mass Media

A mass media approach entails the development of IEC (information, education and communication) materials and their dissemination to the general population through a variety of media channels. The strategy can be implemented through one or several individual campaigns. Determining the strategy here is restricted to campaigns that achieve a high reach of the general population or large sub-groups such as 'the young'. Campaigns focussed on high-risk groups or advertising associated with specific commercial products are not included. Issues relating to these two areas are raised in the sections on sex worker peer education, condom social marketing and prevention strategies among injecting drug users. Also excluded here is use of the press through passing AIDS news to journalists. This can add to the efforts used by other mass media.

The objectives of most AIDS-associated mass media campaigns are:

(a) to disseminate information, raise awareness and stimulate discussion;
(b) to inform people about the availability of more information and services;
(c) to initiate behaviour change to alleviate the risk of infection, usually through increased condom use; minimum number of sexual partners; and reduced incidence of sex with high-risk partners;
(d) to reduce misconceptions about casual transmission; and
(c) to prevent discrimination against those infected with HIV.

The first three of these are of importance here with respect to HIV prevention. The difficulty of using mass media directed at the general population is to develop messages that are easily understands acceptable and personally persuasive. The strategy has the potential to reach a large number of people relatively easily. Its reach depends on the form of media used and access to that media amongst the groups targeted. In most of the countries where AIDS has been reported, the government has taken some steps to inform people about the risks and prevention of the disease. The extent and way in which media is used is very varied. Initial campaigns were fast developed in response to HIV and were typically ill prepared. Later on campaigns were more suited for their respective circumstances, had specific aims, and focused on particular audiences. This was got through more careful planning, such as using focus group discussions and market research to define the issues that needed attention, and then testing, revising and re-testing messages with prospective audiences and key interest groups to ascertain their clarity, appropriateness and acceptability and to prevent any negative side effects.

Description of Potential Projects

There are different ways in which mass media campaigns are conducted - their intensity, level of coverage, quality and the type(s) of media used. The media used include radio, television, film, music, entertainment, news-papers, journals, posters, pamphlets and stickers. In developed countries, more use has been made of television and newspapers to get high levels of IEC coverage. Some countries have added these strategies with household distribution of information brochures. Developing countries have tended to focus on radio and printed materials distributed through a number of outlets such as clinics, schools and public transport. Government mass media campaigns have mostly used broadcast and print media channels whereas local groups have focused on print media and personal contact.

In any one country, there are often many HIV prevention strategies running at one time. and the boundaries of a mass media strategy vis-a-vis other strategies, such as social marketing or AIDS education in schools, may not be clear. To a certain extent, the boundaries are false due to the synergy between the different strategies. For example, a government mass media campaign may increase the success of a social marketing organisation and that organisation may popularize and strenthen the messages that the government advertising campaign is imparting. In this way the two strategies are reinforcing and cross-subsidizing each other. In the same way, the effectiveness of a mass media campaign with focus on condom use will be dependent, amongst other things, on the availability and accessibility of condoms provided through other strategies. The effects of person-to-person education strategies may also be reinforced by mass media campaigns.

Variables which Affect Costs

Some of the variables affecting costs are as follows:

(a) *Materials development:* The quantity of time and type of work spent in development of the IEC materials will effect costs. For instance external consultancy resources may be used during this phase. These costs may decrease if the materials used had already been produced elsewhere. For example, material such as films or educational programmes can be purchased from other countries, or material that has already been screened can be re-broadcast.

(b) *Type of media used:* There are clearly different costs related with broadcast media and, for example, print media.

(c) *Intensity of media use:* For example, the length of a programme or publication, how often it is transmitted, and the duration of the campaign.

(d) *Quality of the media:* For instance, whether peak or off-peak hours are used for broadcasting.

(e) *Rate of charging for airtime or press space:* The expenses of media coverage may be paid for at commercial rates, or sponsored by the private sector, or subsidized by the government.

(f) *Economies of scale:* Mass media campaigns generally have high fixed costs. Therefore, the larger the population and the greater the population density, the lower are likely to be mass media unit costs. Conversely, the smaller the population and the widespread it is will make it more expensive per person covered.

(g) *Country variation in the costs of media production and transmission:* The variations can be sizeable, and make international comparisons between projects difficult.

AIDS Education in Schools

Objectives

AIDS education in schools is a specialized type of IEC (information, education and communication) programme, carried out by teachers and other school staff. It is assumed that the strategy is implemented during school time. It will normally be implemented after development of a school curriculum for AIDS education and will be mostly disseminated in wider sex education activities. The objectives of AIDS school eduction programmes will be similar to those of mass media programmes including:

(a) to provide information, raise awareness and initiate discussion;

(b) to encourage the development of safe behaviour to minimize the vulnerability of infection through, for example, delayed first intercourse or increased condom use;

(c) to correct disinformation about casual transmission; and

(d) to prevent discrimination against those infected with HIV.

Like in other mass media strategies, resources will initially be used in the development and production of education materials aimed at school children. The type of media used will generally be printed materials for use in the classroom (readers, activity sheets, booklets for students, teaching guides for teachers), but videos, posters and magazines may also be produced.

School education programmes are more labour-intensive, utilizing a variety of school staff and students to deliver AIDS education. Staff involved may include school teachers and school counsellors. Head teachers may be given training to make them appreciate the importance of AIDS education in their schools. In the absence of this sensitization, trained teachers may be stopped from implementing the strategy because of resistance from their colleagues. Schools have the capacity to raise awareness and influence both short- and long-term behaviour because they provide an environment where children and young adults are initiated learn and to respond to authority. It is generally thought that the target population is not infected and that the benefits of the strategy will show up some time after its implementation through improved knowledge, attitudes and behaviour. AIDS education in schools is likely to be carried out as a discrete programme. Potential benefits of the programme may, however, be strengthened by other complementary strategies, such as mass media campaigns aimed at the general population or young adolescents, condom social marketing projects and other projects that increase condom availability.

Description of Programmes

AIDS schools education programmes are generally implemented in the government sector, through additions to the school syllabus. A programme may be implemented nationally or reach may be more restricted, for instance, to a regional or municipal initiative. A programme may include partnership with other agencies such as NGOs running smaller-scale school education projects. The acceptability of an AIDS school education programme and its content will rely highly on the cultural context and therefore will differ a great deal between countries. Programmes will also differ with respect to their quality and intensity. For example, a programme may involve only a brief training session for teachers followed by one-off sessions with children during which message are relayed and materials handed out. There may also be AIDS education incorporated into the national curriculum, where teachers may receive several weeks' training, and children may have regular classes over several years. These classes may combine AIDS education with more general health and sex education and use a numbers of participatory approaches to discuss HIV and promote healthy sexual behaviour.

Variables which Affect Costs

Some of the variables affecting unit costs are as follows:

(a) *Development of educational materials:* the amount of time and type of work spent in development of AIDS school curricula and supporting materials. For instance, external consultancy resources may or may not be hired during this phase.

(b) *Production of educational materials:* the quantity and quality of educational materials produced for each student and teacher covered by the strategy.

(c) *Training school teachers:* the amount of time spent in sensitization and training of school staff.

(d) *The amount of school teaching time dedicated to AIDS education.*

(e) *Personnel costs:* the strategy is labour-intensive and the relative costs of trainers and teachers should be kept in mind white making any international comparisons.

(f) *Economies of scale:* the larger the target population, the greater the strategy's fixed overhead costs, such as costs of curricula and material development, will be distributed over more schools and schoolchildren, thus bringing down unit costs.

Social Marketing of Condoms

'Social Marketing' is the marketing of public health goods or ideas through conventional marketing channels. Condom social marketing (CSM) was initially started as part of contraceptive social marketing which has ever since developed as a strategy for the prevention of AIDS. This is due to its potential to distribute large numbers of condoms. Condoms are one of the main ways in which individuals can protect themselves from HIV infection, as well as from other STDs that may facilitate HIV transmission during subsequent exposure to the infection. Enhancing reach of condoms or its complements are an important part of the majority of the other strategies discussed here. In many countries, people cannot get condoms readily, regularly or cheaply. Condoms may not be easily available at a time suitable to consumers. They tend to sell for a relatively high price in the commercial sector or be distributed freely or at a small fee through the public sector. In the former situation, price can present access for many potential users, in the latter situation, condom quality is often low, or thought to be so, and availability may be irregular. The main objective of CSM projects is to increase the availability and use of good-quality, low-cost condoms and thus help is preventing the transmission of HIV infection.

The strategy generally promotes condom use and use of the social marketing organisation's own condom brand in particular. The strategy also aims to spread information concerning HIV prevention, safe sexual behaviour and correct condom use. These goals are achieved through fairly standard marketing techniques with the main activities consisting of conducting market research to acquiring and package condoms; advertising and promoting the product; training retailers; distributing the product; managing the project. The non-clinical nature of condoms enables a wide range of potential retailers, including health professionals, pharmacists, midwives, traditional birth attendants, traditional healers, shopkeepers and itinerant salesmen to participate in the project. Condoms can be sold in both traditional outlets (e.g. pharmacies) and non-traditional outlets (e.g. petrol stations, hotels). In practice, a variety of means of distribution have been developed to ascertain high coverage. Project activities are designed according to the context and environment in which the strategy is being launched. Social marketing projects can inspire demand for condoms by conducting market research and then launching appropriate promotion and advertising campaigns. These may be similar to the mass media campaigns discussed above, but emphasize more on target groups and relying on local promotions as well as on the wider coverage achieved through mass media.

Once demand is initiated commercial companies may themselves be prepared to invest directly in the condom market. Where demand already exists and has clear scope of rising, social marketing has a role to play in increasing the supply of condoms and increasing access through strengthened distribution networks. Although social marketing endeavours to keep condom prices low, some projects launch a variety of condoms to appeal to different parts of the market. In this way, revenue from more expensive condoms can be utilized to cross-subsidize condoms at the lower end of the market. Revenue collected from sales offsets programme costs and reduces the subsidy needed for project activities. The balance struck between cost recovery and demand will to some degree a political decision, denoting the relative importance given to sustainability and coverage.

The costs of many social marketing projects are subsidized by governments or donors, contributing to lower prices and increased access to condoms. In contrast, some projects have accomplished complete self-sufficiency, continuing marketing activities without donor financing or any technical assistance. An example is the Indonesian DauLima Red condom project where commercial partners cover all costs. Large-scale CSM projects are generally taken care or implemented by private not-for-profit organisations. The expertise for these projects has tended to come from a small number of American organisations, either directly or through their subsidiary in-country organisations.

Description of Potential Projects

There are many potential project designs, depending upon the environment in which a project is launched and the varying focus on sustainability and coverage of the implementing organisations. Cisek and Maher (1992) have divided the approaches into four types, with increasing degrees of private sector participation.

Type 1 projects increase availability of condoms by distributing donated supplies. The projects often set up and manage their own administrative structures, implementing agencies and distribution networks. Condoms are largely subsidized and hence within reach of all if distribution networks are adequate. These projects tend to be costly for the donor financing them and tend to remain donor-dependent.

Type 2 projects use available private and public infrastructure to a large extent. For example, a project may arrange for local distributors to conduct distribution and training activities. There is enhanced cost recovery to cover project costs.

Type 3 projects diversify commodity sourcing and are not dependent on donated products. One approach for obtaining condoms is for a project to negotiate reduced prices with condom manufacturers. In return for this donor funds are used for promotion and marketing of these products, in effect running specialized IEC campaigns on the manufacturer's behalf. This may be the most suitable approach in countries where demand is less and potential manufacturers are apprehensive about investing in market development themselves. This type of project would utilize the existing distribution network and contribute to its development.

Type 4 projects maximize the use of private sector infrastructures, including commercial sector management of the project. Donors' participation is in market-building but the commercial partners may also contribute to this. The projects have no management costs and no commodity costs. Condoms are sold at a price which covers all costs including profit margins for the private sector distributors, wholesalers and retailers.

Variables which Affect Costs

Some of the variables affecting costs are described as follows:

(a) *Time span of the project:* Start-up costs are generally high, due to the need for market research and product development. This stage often includes a high level of technical support that contributes to the high cost. In addition, the longer the project runs, the more sales will grow, which will result in lowering of unit costs over time.

(b) *Economies of scale:* These depend on the size of the market.
(c) *The nature of the targeted population:* The distribution of the population between rural and urban areas will affect costs.
(d) *The source of obtaining project condoms:* These may be donated to the project, purchased from the international market, or put on to the market at negotiated prices by commercial manufacturers.
(e) *The social marketing model used:* Costs will be effected by the role of the commercial sector in activities such as administration, management, training, promotion and distribution. A Type 1 model will have more costly distribution systems than a Type 4 model. The degree to which the involvement of the commercial sector affects cost will depend on the approach of the costing exercise. If the strategy is of public sector costs only, involvement of the private sector will greatly reduce costs. If the approach is of all providers, costs may decline slightly as it may be more efficient for the private sector to take on these roles than for a social marketing organisation to set up duplicate systems.
(f) *Levels of cost-recovery:* These will affect net project costs.
(g) *Whether or not the main implementing agency only markets condoms:* If other commodities (such as other types of contraceptives) are marketed as well, overhead costs can be shared through the social marketing of a number of commodities.
(h) *Variables that affect the promotion and advertising component of the strategy:* These comprize of what forms of media are actually available to market condoms.

Treatment of Sexually Transmitted Diseases

Sexually, Transmitted Diseases (in the context of this study, curable STD i.e. not including HIV) are a major health problem in developing countries. Over and Piot (1993) point out that they are one of the ten main health problems responsible for loss of healthy life years. As an important cause of morbidity, there would appear to be a strong case for the provision of STD treatment, and this case is reinforced when the interaction between STD and HIV is considered. Unprotected sexual intercourse is a risk factor for both and there are a number of consequences the interaction between the two. HIV infection, through its effect on the immune system, can increase chances of getting STD and also decrease the effectiveness of any STD treatment. In turn, STD can facilitate transmission of HIV, specially in infections where there is genital ulceration. This latter fact indicates the value of treating STD as a means of reducing the risk of HIV transmission, as well as of curing the STD themselves and preventing their further transmission. Here we focus primarily on management of STD. This comprises of the treatment of the disease as well as health education and promotion activities such as counselling, education and condom distribution. Preventive strategies for both STD and HIV will be same as risk factors and target populations are alike. Some of the issues concerning prevention of STD and AIDS in a target group are addressed in the discussion about commercial sex worker peer education. One of the first steps in acting on the basis of strategy should be to develop and disseminate standard STD diagnostic and treatment protocols. Teaching their through seminars, workshops and training sessions is followed by regular supervision of clinicians treating STD.

Additionally, training in areas such as drug supply logistics, counselling and partner notification might increase non-clinical skills. Treatment of patients is likely to include diagnosis by clinical examination and, if available, by laboratory microscopy, blood tests and culture techniques. Diagnosis is difficult for most STD symptoms and especially in women.

As microscopic examination is often not sufficient for diagnosis, and laboratory tests are costly and technically demanding, there is increasing use of medical examination and clinical algorithms for diagnosis (syndromic case management). The syndromic approach uses algorithms based on commonly presenting signs and symptoms to diagnose and treat. Diagnosis is followed by prescription of drugs. Patients should also be counselled and supplied with condoms as an integral part of their management to prevent themselves and their partners from getting further infections. Promotion of condoms is undertaken alongwith some of the other strategies addressed in this document — specially social marketing of condoms, mass media education and sex worker peer education.

Some projects may also include partner notification. This is a form of targeting as here the object is to identify and treat the infector and any infectees of the patient. In this way, the uninfected can protect themselves, the infected can be cured and the patient may be able to prevent himself from becoming re-infected. The service provider or the patient may take responsibility for notifying and referring partners. This outreach service takes up high levels of resources and its feasibility and effectiveness relies upon the cultural environment of the strategy. Wider advantage of the strategy, apart from the reduced spread of HIV, should also be identified. These include reduced morbidity and mortality from STD in general, through STD treatment and increased condom use, and the possibility of preventing unwanted pregnancies through increased use of condoms. There may also be organisational benefits such as increased drug supply systems and reduced costs through adoption of more rational prescribing procedures.

Description of Potential Projects

Projects will differ according to which of the above activities are actually being implemented. The simplest projects may only diagnose and provide drug prescriptions. Other activities such as initiation of treatment protocols, training, counselling, condom provision and partner notification may be seen as optional extras and acted upon according to the motivation and the resources within individual projects. Some STD treatment projects may have a long history excluding AIDS concerns; others may be newly set up or strengthened to make STD treatment more within reach and to affect AIDS transmission. STD treatment projects that are exclusively part of a policy-driven strategy are likely to be in the government sector. Private sector STD treatment facilities are generally set up opportunistically, with profit rather than policy as the main motive. Costing of these enterprises may provide useful information for public sector policy decisions. Some projects could be set up by universities or research groups as operational research projects. This implies that they incur additional costs compared with regular service delivery. The character and level of these costs should be reported in the results of the costing exercise.

If some of the costs would not be incurred in project replication, or are not relevant to project efficiency (e.g. research costs), it may be needed to exclude them from any cost analysis. Differences will also be seen in the way that STD treatment services relate to other parts of the health service. They may be established 'horizontally', signifying that they are integrated with primary health care services for the general population. STD patients may, for instance, be investigated in general outpatient clinics. They may also be established 'vertically', indicating that they are complementary to general primary health care services but established separately from them. In this situation, patients may be investigated specially designated STD clinics. A third option is that STD treatment services may be provided as part of projects that specifically focus on high-risk groups such as sex workers or their clients. Such groups can be expensive to reach with STD treatment services, but the projects may be more cost-effective than other options because of the number of HIV transmissions that they can prevent.

Finally, referral mechanisms may differ between projects. Government STD clinics are likely to refer upwards to their own facilities. Where they exist, private and NGO clinics will refer to secondary and tertiary facilities within their own sector. They may also have arrangements to refer to government facilities.

Variables which Affect Costs

Some of the variables affecting costs are as follows:

(a) *The incidence and occurrence of STD in the general population:* This affects utilization of services and thus unit costs.

(b) *Diagnostic approach:* Whether diagnosis is determined through clinical examination, microscopy or laboratory test, culture or syndromic case management affects costs.

(c) *The sensitivity and specificity of diagnostic procedures:* These procedures may lead to unsuitable or unnecessary treatment.

(d) *Whether drugs are provided by the project:* Drugs could just be prescribed only, with the costs falling on patients.

(e) *The costs of drugs and diagnostic tests:* These are affected by whether they are purchased locally or are imported using foreign exchange.

(f) *The source of project condoms:* These may be purchased from the international market or donated to the project at inflated or subsidized prices.

(g) *The appropriateness of prescribing practices.*

(h) *The activities provided:* Which activities (e.g. development and distribution of standard protocols, partner notification) are actually undertaken in a particular project and to what extent.

(i) *The costs of salaries:* These may involve a high proportion of total costs since the strategy is labour-intensive, involving one-to-one consultation. The relative costs of personnel should be kept in mind in making any international comparisons.

Commercial Sex Worker Peer Education

Peer education projects are mostly labour-intensive strategies. If the target population is accessible and/or a high-risk one, then accrued benefits can be higher and the intervention is likely to be more cost-effective. Commercial sex workers (CSWs) are a high-risk group for HIV infection due to their number of sexual partners and as they often have other STD that aggravate HIV transmission. They therefore tend to be a high-frequency HIV transmitter core group for the rest of the population. Identifying and reaching CSWs in a given population may at the outset be quite time-consuming. Experience has shown that CSWs peer educators can be used beneficially to locate other CSWs and to conduct peer education. It is perceived that working CSWs are more responsive to learning and adopting behaviour change when approached by peers.

The main aims of a peer education project are to encourage CSWs to use condoms with all partners and to go for STD treatment promptly. The CSW peer educator projects may also focus on the CSW clients for educational activities. The projects are mostly managed and implemented by nongovernmental organisations (NGOs). Initial strategy activities include development and production of targeted IEC materials and recruitment and training of CSW peer educators. Most of CSWs are women and projects often engage women who are current or former CSWs to reach them. Once the project is going on typical outreach activities include eduction, skills training (for negotiating with sexual partners and using condoms) and condom sales/distribution. Peer educators can be a successful link between CSWs and STD services, inspiring CSWs and clients to seek screening and treatment.

The activities of a CSW peer education project overlap, or are complementary to, a number of the other strategies addressed in this study, including condom social marketing, mass media education and treatment of STD. The success of the peer education strategy may be partially affected by these other strategies and, in turn, CSW peer educators can play an important role in increasing STD/HIV awareness and increasing condom use. Some of the non-AIDS benefits of this strategy, such as reduced STD prevalence and incidence, and possibly a fall in number of unwanted pregnancies through condom use, should be described when the costing results are presented.

Description of potential projects

The nature of projects implemented generally vary. Facilities where the projects are implemented can include bars, social centres, residences, STD clinics, brothels and truck stops. Educational sessions may be held on a one-to-one basis or organized as group sessions. Peer educators may be employed in formal activities (e.g. educational sessions arranged beforehand) as well as informal activities (such as mentioning HIV/STD transmission when negotiating the price with the client). IEC materials may or may not be used. If used, they may consist of simple pamphlets, comics and posters, to promotional materials such as T-shirts and bags, and specially produced videos and films. Condoms may be distributed freely or sold as part of cost recovery or a commercial enterprise. Peer CSWs involved in the project may be volunteers or salaried staff. The success of these projects depends on the ability of peer educators of mix freely in the community. Using volunteers can substantially decrease the financial cost implementing the project. This cost saving does, however, need to be weighed against high drop-out rates seen amongst volunteers who may not always be able to give priority to project work.

Variables which affect costs

Some of the variables affecting costs are as follows:

(a) *Time and type of work invested in development of appropriate IEC materials.* For instance, external consultancy resources may or may not be used during this phase. IEC materials may also be periodically changed.
(b) *The amount of time invested in staff and peer educator training.*
(c) *The geographical and social accessibility of target groups.*
(d) *The total number of CSWs targeted.*
(e) *Whether educational sessions between peer educators and CSWs are conducted with individuals or groups.*
(f) *Whether peer educators are salaried or voluntary staff.*
(g) *Types of educational materials used in the sessions.*
(h) *The source of getting the project condoms.*

Voluntary Counselling and Testing

HIV voluntary counselling testing (VCT) plays a big role in HIV prevention activities. VCT has received more importance due to the increasing profile of interventions to prevent mother-to-child transmission and options for care and management of opportunistic infections (e.g. preventive therapy for tuberculosis). As part of the counselling measures, VCT can help inform uninfected clients of the risks of HIV and teach HIV-positive people about dealing with and preventing transmission to their partners. However, the implementation of VCT is tedious. A key issue has been the acceptability of VCT and people's readiness to be tested and then return for their results. In Cote d'lvoire, only 17.5 per cent of the HIV-positive women who were initially identified participated in a trial—some were not willing to be tested others did not return for results, and more than 40 per cent refused to enrol in the trial despite being HIV-positive and pregnant. Implementation is better if efforts are made to emphasize on the programmes' process. The hiring of VCT services is low even in well-resourced countries and highlights the role of fear and stigmatization as a barrier to use of these services.

A service providing VCT includes pre-test counselling, post-test counselling, and the test itself. Necessary support activities comprise of training of staff and development and distribution of IEC materials. Counselling should be part of any service that involves testing for HIV. The objectives of VCT are as follows:

(a) to instil motivation to change sexual and drug behaviours. So as to enable seronegative people to protect themselves from infection, and to prevent transmission from seropositive people;

(b) to encourage those vulnerable to high risk to come forward for testing;

(c) to allow early detection of medical and social needs of HIV-infected people, and ascertain that common infections are properly treated;

(d) to enable women to make informed decisions about reproductive health issues;

(e) to facilitate people to deal with stress about HIV-related problems and relieve anxiety associated with uncertainty about HIV serostatus;

(f) to provide a service, including counselling, to those who want to be aware of their serostatus so that they can protect themselves and others from infection and plan for the future.

The main activities of VCT consist of:

(i) A pre-test counselling session, between a trained counsellor and a client, couple or group;

(ii) Laboratory tests, for those clients who wish to go ahead with the test;

(iii) A post-test counselling session for those who have been tested.

There is dispute over the success of VCT at both the individual and population levels: evidence has been reviewed by De Zoysa et al. (1995). A review of 50 studies showed mixed results for the effect of counselling and testing on risky behaviour. A study in Rwanda pointed out increases in reported condom use. Large increases in condom use and refraining followed by successive and intensive counselling among couples found to be discordant (i.e. only one partner infected) in a research project in Zaire. The AIDS Information Centre in Uganda, which provided anonymous HIV testing and counselling, also showed substantial rise in condom use. A study in the United Republic of Tanzania found that a significantly higher proportion of woman than men did not want their spouse to now their HIV status. Although many studies suggest that VCT may be successful, at least in the short term, in improving sexual behaviour amongst heterosexuals and especially when couples are counselled together, the relationship between VCT and a reduction in HIV transmission is complex. One approach that may increase the effectiveness of VCT is the use of rapid testing techniques rather than the widely-used ELISA. This means that people can get results of the same day or relatively quickly.

There has been some concern that VCT, being an expensive option because of its emphasis on personal counselling. It has been suggested that those who choose to take VCT may be a special group, who could perhaps be reached by other, less costly means also. Other non-HIV advantage of VCT that should be reported in the analysis include diagnosis of STD and prevention of STD infection that may be due to changed sexual behaviour. There are concerns about ill effects including psychological pressure, stigmatization, disruption in couple and family relationships, violence and divorce, which causes peoples reluctance to both undergo tests and return for the result. Failures to maintain secrecy may lead to social or work discrimination.

Currently, there is very little information available on the relative costs and effectiveness of the different models of VCT this could help organisations choose between different models.

Description of Potential Projects

VCT is often given by NGOs as well as by government health services, thus making the nature of the services provided quite diverse. The service may be provided as a free-standing project, or may be merged into other services (e.g. antenatal clinics, STD clinics, drug treatment centres, HIV support groups, blood transfusion services). The clinic may intentionally offer an anonymous service to alleviate the risks of discrimination, or its activities may integrated closely to the provision of other health services. The targeted population may be the general population, or special high-risk groups. VCT is now also being carried out by the private sector.

Variables which Affect Costs

These include:

(a) *The geographical and social accessibility of the population.*
(b) *HIV prevalence:* As prevalence rises, the costs of testing will increase, although economies of scale work simultaneously.
(c) *Whether or not particular groups are intentionally encouraged to come for testing.*
(d) *The level of training of counsellors.*
(e) *The degree of emphasis placed on careful and intensive counselling:* In a study in the United Kingdom of HIV testing in antenatal clinics, over 80 per cent of the costs were associated with the time required to ensure that informed consent was given.
(f) *The number attending dependant on the capacity of the service.*
(g) *The type of test and number of tests.*
(h) *The relative importance of the use of volunteers.*
(i) *The relative sophistication of the educational materials used.*
(j) *Whether or not free supplies (e.g. condoms) are distributed, and the source of condoms.*

Prevention Measures Among Injecting Drug Users

Injecting drug users (IDUs) are generally at high risk of HIV infection due to the risk of HIV transmission associated with sharing injecting needless with others. The rapid increase of HIV among IDUs has now been enumerated in an increasing number of countries including countries in Eastern Europe, Latin America and Asia. The incidence of HIV has grown among IDUs and their sexual partners. Vulnerable groups to IDU use comprise of the urban poor, street children, prisoners, sex workers, itinerant and guest workers and communities in drug-producing areas. The major risk factor associated with transmission of HIV among IDUs is multiperson reuse or sharing of syringes. Alongwith this, indirect sharing of equipment such as water, cotton, cookers and other drug preparation equipment has also been the cause of the transmission of HIV. Thus one key objective of IDU interventions is to prevent multiperson reuse of syringes and enable IDUs access to sterile syringes. IDUs are also at high risk from transmission of other bloodborne infections such as hepatitis B and C. The most successful way to prevent HIV transmission among IDUs is the elimination of drug use. However, in reality, programmes work towards alleviating or reducing harm. Thus there is a series of activities and educational messages used: (a) stop using and injecting drugs; (b) if continuing to use drugs, do not share equipment, but use own supplies; (c) if sharing, then disinfect to reduce transmission. The general aim of HIV prevention activities are to increase protective behaviour and reduce risk of HIV infection. This comprise of changing drug use, needle practices and sexual behaviours simultaneously. The HIV prevention strategies for IDUs are highly focussed.

A comprehensive strategy for HIV prevention among IDUs includes:

(a) primary prevention of drug abuse;
(b) disseminating of information, education, counselling to minimize needle/syringe sharing;
(c) use of bleach to clean/disinfect syringes/needles and drug preparation equipment;
(d) changing laws to allow legal buying of needle/syringe, outreach programmes for IDUs, syringe/needle exchange activities;
(e) referral for treatment of health problems such as STD, peer education programmes;
(f) access to substance abuse treatment.

Educational information is disseminated to promote the one-time use of sterile syringes/needles and their safe disposal. IDU programmes are relatively labour-intensive, employing a variety of staff and volunteers. There are many interventions and many outcomes. In presenting the costs of the IDU prevention strategy, the direct and indirect benefits of the strategy should also be documented. Currently, there is very little information available on the costs of the different models of HIV prevention for IDUs in a developing or transitional country context. Based on the limited information, projects promoting access to sterile syringes are relatively cost-effective, especially when compared to the lifetime cost of HIV treatment with respect to United States.

Description of Potential Projects

The characteristics of IDU projects is variable and one of the first tasks of a costing exercise will be to describe the particular project to be costed. HIV prevention activities can occur together with other health services or may be run independently. They often run on a relatively small-scale basis at the community or city level. In general, IDU activities are likely to be carried out as a discrete or stand-alone programme, separate from other HIV prevention strategies focussed at the general population, although there may be complementary strategies such as condom social marketing or distribution and STD treatment.

Type 1 projects are community-based outreach projects and are meant to reach the IDUs' sexual partners and drug-using networks. With the help of community and IDU peer workers, these programmes include activities such as educational messages for risk reduction, bleach distribution, HIV counselling and testing, treatment referrals, condom distribution, as well as trying to change set habits related to unsafe drug use and risky sexual behaviours.

Type 2 projects, needle-exchange programmes (NEPs), provide sterile needles and syringes to IDUs in return of used needles and syringes. Activities include exchange of potentially contaminated syringes, bleach distribution, treatment referrals, condom distribution, educational messages for risk education, HIV testing and counselling and screening for other infectious diseases.

Type 3 projects focus on drug abuse treatment. They aim to eliminate and decrease drug use through replacement use of illegal drugs with substances like methadone. These programmes may comprize individual and group counselling, HIV testing and counselling and referrals to other health care services, as well as educational messages to reduce risky drug use and sexual behaviour.

Type 4 projects try to affect risky behaviour by changing the pattern of drug use and sexual networks through network-style interventions. This is done through the use of IDU peers who may be seen as opinion leaders in their networks.

These activities may be accompanied by media interventions such as television, radio and newspaper advertisements promoting the main educational messages as well as the intervention. Community-based outreach programmes are generally used in places where NEPs are not viable legally. There have also been attempts to involve pharmacists in the sale, distribution, or exchange of syringes in Europe, North America and Asia. Pharmacy-based programmes often give IDUs a choice of prepared packs. Pharmacy-based activities have lower initial costs because there is already an established distribution network. Other advantages to pharmacy-based interventions are their accessibility geographically, with longer opening hours. Using volunteers can substantially reduce the financial cost of implementing the project. This cost saving does, however, need to be weighed against high drop-out rates seen amongst volunteers who may not always be able to give priority to project work. Initial strategy activities consist of development and production of targeted IEC materials and recruitment and training of IDU volunteers/peers. Once the project is on typical outreach activities comprise of distribution of educational materials, peer education, and the distribution and exchange of supplies.

Factors which Affect Costs

Key intervention-related factors, which will affect the level of costs, are:

(a) *Nature of activities and integration with other services.*
(b) *Materials development:* The amount of time and type of work invested in development of the IEC materials will influence costs.
(c) *The amount of time invested in staff and peer educator training.*
(d) *The geographical and social accessibility of target groups.*
(e) *The total number of IDUs targeted:* Large numbers imply greater expenditure on some of the IEC materials and on supplies but may contribute to lower average costs.
(f) *The intensity of contact between peer educators and IDUs:* Whether educational sessions are conducted with individuals or groups.

(g) *Whether peer educators are salaried or voluntary staff.*

(h) *Type, intensity and quality of media used:* There are clearly different costs associated with broadcast media and, for example, print media relative to radio and television. The length, frequency, duration as well as peak or off-peak air time of programmes also affect cost.

(i) *Rate of charging for airtime or press space:* May be paid for at commercial rates, or sponsored by the private sector, or subsidized by the government.

(j) *Personnel costs:* The strategy is labour-intensive and the relative costs of staff should be borne in mind in making any international comparisons.

(k) *Provision of project condoms:* May be bought on the international market or donated to the project at inflated or subsidized prices.

(l) *Whether drugs are provided by the project:* Alternatively, they may be prescribed only, the costs falling on patients.

(m) *The existence of complementary activities:* Like legal and welfare counselling.

Prevention of Mother-To-Child/Vertical Transmission

The risk of vertical transmission from an infected mother to her baby ranges from 21 per cent to 43 per cent in developing countries, contingent on the breastfeeding patterns. The virus may be transmitted during pregnancy (*in utero*), childbirth (*intra-partum*), or through breastfeeding (*post-partum*). The primary strategy for preventing vertical transmission is avoiding HIV infection in girls and women. However, there are several ways known to be effective during pregnancy, childbirth and post-natally to lower the risk of transmission from an HIV-positive mother to her baby. The key interventions for prevention of mother-to-child transmission (MTCT), are as follows:

(i) Antiretroviral (ARV) Therapies

Transmission to the baby can be reduced by two-thirds with the administration of long-course Antiretroviral therapy with zidovudine (ZDV). The administration of this medicine is complex and costly. Several clinical trials have examined shorter and cheaper

ARV regimens. The success of the Thai short-course trial in reducing MTCT by 50 per cent among a non-breastfeeding population led to more emphasis on non-breastfeeding strategies in developing countries. Studies among breastfeeding populations find a 38-44 per cent reduction in MTCT using a short-course ZDV regimen. In 1999, a Ugandan clinical trial found that a single dose of nevirapine (NVP) taken during labour ad by the infant after birth was almost 50 per cent more successful than the short-course ZDV regimen.

(ii) Provision and Advice on Infant Feeding

The success of ARV therapy in these clinical trials, there is increasing emphasis on infant feeding and MTCT in developing countries. It is observed that breastfeeding doubles the transmission of HIV. Factors that increase the risk of transmission include longer span of breastfeeding and the stage of infectivity. Observations from one trial show that exclusively breastfed infants were less likely to become infected than non-breastfed or mixed-fed infants. It is not clear how the duration of breastfeeding and early weaning affect these results. MTCT through breastfeeding has become a very important source of debate, given the intensive efforts on the part of both national and international communities to advocate for breastfeeding over the past 20 years. There are major concerns regarding the use of formula feeding leading to increased sickness/ mortality of infants, and other feeding choices such as early weaning, surrogate breastfeeding and pasteurization of breast milk.

There is concern about the difficult formula of pasteurization, and there have been cases where surrogate mothers have acquired the HIV infection from infected infants. VCT (Voluntary Counselling and Testing) has also received increased attention due to the high profile of MTCT prevention. Given the success of the ARV interventions, there have been several studies related to the cost-effectiveness of MTCT prevention interventions. But, there is limited information on the cost of implementing such work outside a trial context. In general, the cost of the intervention has been deduced by mixing data from a number of sources and countries. While this method can guide priority-setting in a global context, it is difficult to infer costs and resource requirements. The emphasis of analysis has been mainly on the cost of ARV drugs, and there have been only a few attempts made to model the infrastructure needs for such an intervention. It is necessary to consider what extra infrastructure and staff are required and also where they might come from. There is very restricted cost information on the provision and distribution of formula feeding for the infants of HIV-positive women, and the expenses of using replacement methods for HIV-positive women as well as their families.

Description of Potential Projects

The setting up of MTCT prevention interventions is still in its initial phases in many countries. Testing and offering of anti-retrovirals generally occur within the existing health and antenatal care infrastructure. The actual timing of the HIV testing and counselling depends on the nature of regimen that is being undertaken and the stage of pregnancy at which a woman first attends antenatal services. There are major problems associated with women consenting to and then coming back for HIV test results, before undertaking antiretroviral therapy (as discussed in the VCT strategy). Different models of VCT and feeding advice are currently being assimilated.

Variables which Affect Costs

Key issues affecting costs are as follows:

(a) *Antiretroviral regimen:* The choice and price of drugs significantly affect the costs of the intervention.
(b) *HIV prevalence:* The costs of testing and delivery of the regimen will increase as prevalence rises. Though economies of scale are also observed.
(c) *Extent of additional capacity which is needed to administer the regimen:* Existing facilities and services may require to be strengthened.
(d) *Feeding methods:* Provision of replacement feeding methods, such as formula-milk, will significantly increase costs.
(e) *The geographical and social reach of the population.*
(f) *The numbers attending relative to the capacity of the service.*
(g) *The type of test and number of tests.*

Emerging HIV Prevention Strategies

Apart from the already established strategies being implemented, at present there are also new and emerging HIV prevention strategies. Which are in different stages of development and clinical trials, and the feasibility of their use in a low- and middle-income country context is still being found out.

These emerging strategies include: (a) microbicides and female-controlled methods; and (b) use of vaccines.

Microbicides and Female-controlled Methods

There has been wide spread curiosity in female-controlled methods for prevention of HIV. There are many producers of female condoms, which are actively being marketed through social marketing programmes in several countries. There is also debate about the role of existing spermicides in preventing STD/HIV. The development of chemical barrier methods such as vaginal microbicides to prevent HIV infections is in progress. Both product development, including clinical evaluation, and product acceptability studies are going on. It is not expected that these microbicides will be available for some years. Till now there has been little talk of programmatic issues such as introduction, distribution and post-marketing research as well as analysis of the costs and cost-effectiveness of microbicides. However, it is expected that microbicides would be sold through current contraceptive marketing programmes.

Vaccines

As of now, vaccines for HIV are in the clinical trial stage in the United States and Thailand. There is still controversy whether these clades of the vaccine will be suitable in other settings, e.g. sub-Saharan Africa. Some preliminary modelling on the cost-effectiveness of vaccines has brought out a range of factors that will affect costs.

(a) production costs including fixed costs
(b) implementation costs including
  - training and health education
  - establishing stores/cold chains
(c) programme costs (vaccine, staff, transportation, fixed costs)
  - costs of adverse reactions

Further, the cost-effectiveness of these vaccines will depend on population access (high-risk groups versus general population), the timing of expected effect on HIV incidence, need for booster doses and infectious rate among the target groups.

Eight

Cost Analysis: Fundamentals and Choices

Meaning of Costs

Economists define a cost as the value of resources used to produce a good or service. However, the way these resources are measured may vary. There are two main options with respect to measurement of these resources: financial and economic costing.

Financial costs: These represent actual expenditure on goods and services purchased. Costs are thus described in relation to how much money has been paid for the resources used in the project or service. In order to find out the financial costs of a project, we require to know the price and quantity of all the resources used or, alternatively, the level of expenditure on these goods and services.

Economic costs: Economists ascertain costs in a broader way. They define costs in terms of the alternative uses of resources that have been forgone by using a resource in a particular way. These economic or opportunity costs acknowledge the cost of using resources, as these resources are then unavailable for productive use elsewhere.

"The basic concept is that things have a value that might not be fully included in their price. It is not difficult in many health programmes to recognize resource inputs for which little or no money is paid: volunteers working for free health messages broadcast without charge; vaccines or other supplies donated or provided at a large discount by organisations or individuals". Thus the value of these resources to society, regardless of who pays for them, is measured by opportunity cost.

Economic costs: thus consist of the estimated value of goods or services for which there were no financial transactions or when the price of certain goods did not show the cost of using it productively elsewhere. The main ways that financial and economic costs differ is in the way they treat: (a) donated goods and services; (b) other inputs whose prices are incorrect or distorted; and (c) valuation of capital items.

When to use financial, economic or both approaches depends on the objectives of the analysis. If the aim of the costing exercise is to compare expenditure against budget allocations or to explore affordability of the project, then only actual project expenditure should be recorded. Here, the financial cost of a consumed resource for which nothing was paid, for example a donated good, is zero. But if, the purpose of the costing exercise is to measure the project sustainability or to consider repeating the project elsewhere, the concern will be to record the costs of all resources consumed, whether or not they were paid for from the project budget. Here, the economic costs of donated goods and services, valued by their equivalent market prices, are used in the analysis. "Analyses using economic costs do not replace those using financial costs, but supplement them with additional information useful for decision-making".

Society, Provider, Household and Private Costs

A *societal perspective* would include strategy-related costs incurred by all members of society, including the private sector, the public sector and private consumers (e.g. households and individuals). A *provider perspective* would not include costs incurred by private consumers or households. A public sector perspective would not include costs incurred by the private sector and by private consumers, and include only those costs incurred by the public sector in implementing the strategy. These costs can be understood to be the costs of providing particular programmes, and are borne by the organisation delivering the services (although this does not imply that the organisation finances the entire cost of the services). In addition, individuals and households may also incur costs when using these services.

Apart from providing funds directly through the payment of user fees, private individuals may also contribute to financing service delivery through the provision of goods. For instance, some blood transfusion patients may have to buy their bags and needles privately before coming to the service, and many STD treatment patients will have to buy their drugs privately from pharmacies.

These guidelines help calculate the cost of projects from the service providers perspective and not from the perspective of the society and its individuals. The only portion of the household cost that will be considered is the amount of fees or payments made which contribute towards financing services and will be known as *private costs*. The information regarding fees collected from clients of HIV prevention services can support to the debate on cost recovery. For example, analysis from specific projects can give an idea of the percentage of project running costs that can potentially be covered from fees—an issue that is very important to sustainability of projects and one that is often focused on by donors. Including full household costs implies including a wider range of private costs, such as travel and time costs.

Full and Incremental Cost Analysis

A full cost analysis ascertains the costs of all resources that are used in running a project or programme, including basic infrastructure. An incremental analysis takes into account the cost of adding or implementing the additional project or programme to existing services. It does not attempt to give cost estimates for existing services. An incremental analysis accounts for the major 'new' inputs that are needed by the new intervention. However, since it is known that the organisational infrastructure already exists, an incremental costing will undermine costs that are of a general administrative nature borne by the organisation (particularly communications and office supplies). Similarly, it does not include such as the overhead costs of running the organisation as is done in a full costing analysis. It is also more cumbersome to generalize from incremental cost analyses, unless the prior level of existing services and infrastructure is clearly specified. The incremental approach is particularly suitable to use when the intervention or project is no the major component of the organisation's overall cost structure. The availability and ease of data collection as well as organisational structures may have an impact on whether a full or incremental costing is undertaken.

Total, Average and Marginal Costs

Total cost: represents the cost of producing a quantity of services or output for a particular project or programme. This can be the result of a full or incremental cost analysis.

Average cost: is the total cost per unit of output, and is calculated by dividing total cost by the units of output or services produced.

Marginal cost: is the additional cost of producing one more unit of output.

This should not be mixed with incremental costs that consist of the additional cost of adding on an entire service or project, whereas marginal costs are concerned with cost differences within a service or project.

The purpose of the cost analysis will determine whether to focus on average or marginal costs. If you want to look at variations in costs between different providers or clinics, you should compare average costs. If you want to look at the effect of expanding services (e.g. expanding hours or number of staff), then you need to consider marginal costs.

Joint Costs

The resources that you are costing may not be completely utilized the specific project or programme that is being examined (e.g. a person may be working on a number of projects, some not dealing with HIV prevention). They may be used together with other ongoing project. Whereby, a decision needs to be made about what proportion of the resources should be allocated to the specific project or programme that is being costed, and the way it should be apportioned. The way you allocate the resources may vary according to the type of resource, and this will be discussed in chapter 4.

Classification of Costs

"To estimate a health programme's cost, it is necessary to classify its components. Cost elements can be split up in several ways. A good classification scheme depends on the needs of the particular situation, but there are three essential elements: (a) it must be suited to the particular situation; (b) the classes (categories) must not overlap; and (c) the classes selected must cover all possibilities.

"Resources used for programmes can be described in many different ways. For example, an HIV prevention programme might be using the following resources: personnel, money from external sources and mass media. These categories are well defined and their meaning is clear. However, they do not consist of a very useful way of thinking about the resources used in this programme. The main problem is that the categories overlap; money from external source can be utilized to pay for personnel, and personnel are likely to be involved in mass media operations. If we add up the value of these three categories, they may well exceed the total cost of the programme.

Classification of Costs by Inputs

The main type of cost-classification is by inputs, these are considered as either recurrent items (those that are used up in the course of a year and are usually purchased regularly) and capital items (those that last longer than a year).

Capital Costs

(a) Vehicles: bicycles, motorcycles, four-wheel-drive vehicles, trucks
(b) Equipment: refrigerators, sterilizers, manufacturing machinery, scales, other equipment with a unit cost (price) of $100 or more
(c) Buildings, space: health centres, hospitals, training schools, administrative offices, storage facilities
(d) Training, non-recurrent: training activities for personnel that occur once or rarely
(e) Social mobilization activities, non-recurrent: e.g.

promotion, publicity campaigns, that occur only once or rarely

(f) Start-up activities: which are likely to last the lifetime of the project, such as production of materials, recruitment of staff

Recurrent Costs

(a) Personnel (all types): supervisors, administrators, consultants, casual labour and volunteers
(b) Supplies: drugs, vaccines, syringes, educational materials, condoms, small equipment (unit cost less than $100)
(c) Vehicles, operation and maintenance: petrol, diesel, lubricants, tyres, spare parts, registration, insurance
(d) Buildings, operation and maintenance: electricity, water, heating, fuel, telephone, telex, insurance, cleaning, painting, repairs to electrical supply/ appliances, plumbing, roofing and heating
(e) Training, recurrent (e.g. short in-service courses)
(f) Social mobilization: operating costs
(g) Other operating costs not included above

Costs can also be classified according to the following parameters:

(a) function/activity;
(b) organisational level (e.g. national, district, community);
(c) source of funds (e.g. national and local governments, donors, nongovernmental organisations); and
(d) type of currency

HIV Prevention Strategies Outcome Measure

Unit costs are another term for average costs. They can be calculated for both financial and economic cost analysis. For a specific project or programme, several types of unit costs can be calculated, depending on the type of outcome that is specified. The outcomes can be of three types:

(a) Primary outcome, which measures the final effect on health status as an outcome of the project;

(b) Intermediate outcome, which shows the intermediate changes due to the intervention of the project, required before there is a health impact;

(c) Immediate or process measure, which measures the activities or outputs of the intervention.

Problems

For the HIV prevention strategies, the primary outcome measure is the number of HIV infections averted. There are many practical problems in finding the number of HIV infections averted: (1) The most direct method to find the infections averted is by randomized clinical trials, which are both expensive and rarely implemented for behavioural change interventions. (2) In order to calculate the full effect of the intervention, we need to take into account both infections averted for those people involved in the intervention, as well as secondary infections averted because the chain of transmission has been broken. This needs information about the epidemiology behavioural patterns and transmission success in the specific population; (3) If many prevention strategies are being used together; it is hard to attribute infections averted to any specific strategy.

Three ways have been used to overcome these problems:

(1) Other primary outcome measures, such as Disability-Adjusted Life Years (DALYs), have been suggested;

(2) intermediate or process-measures have been used.

Table 1 discusses the strengths and weaknesses of the different measures that have been used in measuring outcomes of HIV prevention strategies. Third, model-based measurement has developed as a means of estimating HIV infections averted. These models aim to capture the dynamic nature of this transmission, as well as epidemiological and behavioural patterns. The models are used to provide simulations about the possible impact of HIV prevention strategies on the total number of HIV infections averted (including secondary infections). The development of the models can be quite difficult.

TABLE 1

THE STRENGTHS AND WEAKNESSES OF DIFFERENT OUTCOME MEASURES

Outcome Measure	*Strengths*	*Weaknesses*
Disability-adjusted life years (DALYs) gained - primary outcome.	• Cross-sector, cross-programme and cross-interventions comparisons are possible. • Ability to assess impact of combined clinical management and prevention strategies. • Morbidity and mortality effects combined in one measure. • Ability to measure consequences of clinical management when death is certain outcome. • Can include indirect consequences such as TB or STD cases treated and/ or prevented.	• Based on subjective measures of disability. • Possible over-simplification. • Derived from and dependent on the primary outcome of the intervention. • Debate over their validity, • Not widely recognized outside the health sector.
Infections averted - primary outcome of an HIV prevention strategy—primary outcome.	• Comparisons across different prevention strategies are possible. • DALYs can be derived easily with adequate information on mortality and life expectancy.	• Unable to evaluate strategies that include clinical management component. • Unable to compare across health interventions. • Unless measured through randomized controlled trials, may need sophisticated modelling to assess impact on general population. • May not include indirect consequences of intervention.

(Contd.)

(Contd.)

Outcome Measure	*Strengths*	*Weaknesses*
Numbers educated or counselled; cases detected through screening for blood transfusions and counselling-intermediate outcome measure,	• Relative ease of measurement and interpretation. • May give some indication of impact, even though final health status unknown. • Reflects operational efficiency of programme. • Can identify most efficient method of delivery.	• No measure of impact on HIV transmission. • Does not account for variations in populations' HIV seroprevalence. • Gain achieved may not reflect real change in impact.
Condoms distributed or sold/numbers receiving educational material; numbers tested/screened - process-outcome measure.	• Ease of collection, these measures are often part of routine monitoring of programmes. • Reflects operational efficiency of programme. • Can identify most efficient method of delivery.	• No measure of impact on HIV transmission. • Does not account for variations in populations' HIV seroprevalence. • Gain achieved may not reflect real change in impact.

Given the differences in outcome measures, there can be a number of unit costs derived for a particular project or programme. For instance, let us assume that the total costs of a peer education project were $30,000 for one year, where there were 1040 education sessions in that year reaching 2496 people. Using a model-based analysis, there is an estimate that there were 250 HIV infections averted (based on information about behavioural changes and increased use of condoms). Then, for this peer education programme among sex workers, the following type of unit costs could be derived:

(i) an immediate service or process (output): cost per education session
= $30,000/1040
= $ 28.85 per education session

(ii) an intermediate effect: cost per person educated
= $ 30,000/2496
= $ 12.01 per person educated

(iii) a final effect or impact on health status: cost per HIV infection averted
= $ 30,000/250
= $ 120 per HIV infection averted

It may be possible to find out unit costs by activity within a project or programme if activity-specific outputs are available (for instance, if we know that training activities cost $5000 and there were 60 people trained, then the cost per person trained is $83.33). In practice, the calculation of the final impact can be quite difficult and relies on the kind of the prevention strategies being considered. For a strategy such as HIV blood screening, it is possible to calculate the cases of HIV infection directly averted. However, to calculate the number of secondary infections requires model-based evaluation or randomized clinical trials. Thus, for most research, process or intermediate unit costs are often presented (e.g. cost per condom distributed, number of people buying condoms). But, it is suggested that the calculation of unit cost should try and use outcome measures that are closer to the health impact end of the spectrum. Thus, for the condom social marketing project, reporting 'costs per condom distributed and reported used' will be more effective terms of extrapolating impact.

Cost-effectiveness

Cost-effectiveness analysis is a tool which facilitates programme managers to make informed decisions about resource allocation. By measuring and comparing the costs and effects of various interventions, their relative efficiency can be measured and future resource requirements estimated. The key feature of cost-effectiveness analysis is that it is used to examine all options that work to meet the same objective. The results of the analysis are described with respect to the cost per unit of effectiveness for each option.

The cost-effectiveness ratio is calculated for each option by dividing cost by the unit of effect (e.g. HIV infection averted). Then a comparison is made between these ratios. The option with the least cost per unit of effectiveness is the most cost-effective, and is likely to be preferred because of economic efficiency. Cost analysis is one of the main building blocks for cost-effectiveness studies. Unit costs based on intermediate outputs can be considered as preliminary cost-effectiveness results; more ambitious cost-effectiveness analyses are focused at health status impacts.

There is a paucity of data on the relative cost-effectiveness of the different prevention strategies that are being implemented around the world. Costing and subsequent cost-effectiveness analysis can contribute to greater awareness in this area and enable decision-making about the best use of present and new resources. For instance, if a country gets a loan or grant for AIDS-related prevention activities, cost-effectiveness data would enable planners to assess which strategies, and what combination and volume of each, might provide the best value for money with respect to the objectives.

Nine

Planning the Costing Analysis

Objectives of Cost Analysis

Analysis of the costs of HIV prevention may be carried out for a number of reasons. Before initiating a costing study, a manager should be clear about the questions s/he is seeking to answer, the object of the planned work and the use to which the work will be put. These will facilitate in establishing the boundaries for the costing exercise. For instance, it should be clear whether the exercise is being conducted to ascertain the costs and efficiency of only on-going activities, or whether it is being conducted with a view to project replicability. If these types of issues are clear at the outset, it will be simpler to ascertain exactly what data are to be collected and there will be less possibility of wasting time in unnecessary activities. Objectives for a cost analysis can include:

(i) Ascertaining the Efficiency of a Project

The objectives of the costing exercise could be to analyse on-going costs of an established project to identify potential cost savings and to modify the efficiency of the service. In this case, project start-up costs may be excluded. Within a project, a manager may need to analyse expenditure by input to know which areas of the programme involve high or low spending. In order to exclude project start-up costs, all work that is undertaken to initiate the project are excluded from the analysis.

(ii) Modification/Sustainability

If the onus to conduct the costing exercise is coming from the project itself, managers may want information for one, or a combination, of the following objectives: improving budgeting; monitoring costs; planning improvement of the current system, and improving the future of the strategy. A manager may, for instance, be particularly concerned about the sustainability of the HIV prevention programme and looking for an accurate estimate of the budget necessary to maintain it. If charging for services is a choice, ·information on costs can help to establish appropriate prices. Cost analysis may also be needed in discussions about the feasibility of scaling-up/expanding the project. If sustainability is the main criteria, start-up costs are excluded, but if one is considering the expansion of a project, then it is necessary to know whether certain aspects of start-up activities need to take place.

(iii) Replication

If the initiative for the costing exercise is coming from outside the project, objectives are more likely to focus on replicability of the project and extrapolation of results to other situations. Local managers may give considerable time to the fieldwork phase and it is necessary that the resulting data also be of use and value to them. This is particularly true with CSM. Most formal CSM projects are managed by foreign private groups of their subsidiaries. These organisations' financial management is generally strong and they will be monitoring costs for their own purposes.

The objective of a costing exercise is, therefore, not likely to be that of collating information on the on-going costs of the project for management purposes, but rather that of finding the costs of this strategy relative to the other main strategies or giving information on costs of replication of the project elsewhere. If the objective is to give information on the total costs of the strategy with a view to replication, both on-going and start-up costs should be collected. Start-up costs comprise any development and production of information, education and communication (IEC) materials as well as dissemination of diagnostic and treatment protocols, IEC, and recruitment of workers.

(iv) Cost-effectiveness

A manager may need more information on the relative cost-effectiveness of alternative ways of delivering the prevention strategy for which s/he is responsible. Cost-effectiveness studies can help in priority setting, resource allocation decisions and design of services. As an example, decisions may require to be made within a sex worker/peer education project on whether to engage part-time volunteer workers or full time salaried staff. Cost analysis may help in understanding the differences between such options, weighing the tension between increased costs and also increased effectiveness, and thus helping in the planning of a new or expanded projects.

Another objective of the costing exercise may be to compare the cost-effectiveness of different HIV prevention strategies relative to each other (e.g. compare school education relative to strategies of CSW peer education). Since alternative delivery channels may be considered, it is necessary to include start-up costs if the objective is to find out the relative cost-effectiveness. There is great difficulty in finding out the effectiveness of mass media campaigns and, particularly, in attributing effects to the campaigns rather than to any other kind of media or information source. It is thus not expected that costs will be studied to compare the relative cost-effectiveness of a mass media campaign with other strategies.

(v) Private/provider perspectives

Whereas the private costs other than fees paid (e.g. for the purchase of condoms) are excluded from the costing analysis; but they should be mentioned in the presentation of the costing data. However, some CSM projects are exclusively in the private sector and will, by definition, have a private provider perspective. Other projects cover the private and public sectors and the focus will depend upon who is commissioning the costing exercise and its objectives. If, for instance, a Ministry of Health wants to find out the financial implications for its own budget of undertaking a CSM project, the cost analysis may be based entirely on public sector expenditure, i.e., the expenditure of the government and donor-funded portion of the project.

Identifying the Most Effective Combination of Strategies

In the earlier portion we have studied the different HIV prevention strategies individually. In practice, however, HIV prevention projects are unlikely to take place in such neatly defined packages. Indeed, it is acknowledged that a combination of approaches can be mutually and positively strengthening. For example, the success of a school education programme or a condom distribution programme may depend on the success of a concurrently running mass media campaign. In the same way, a CSW peer education project may combine STD treatment, counselling and condom promotion. As the boundaries between strategies may not be clear, it is important to be particular about what exactly is being costed, what combination of strategies is being examined, what options are being compared and, if proceeding to undertake cost-effectiveness analysis, what the suitable measures of effect/outcome are for the costs being measured.

For instance, it should be clear at the outset whether the object is to cost one particular mass media campaign or to cost a wider mass media strategy that may include a number of campaigns conducted by one or several organisations. HIV blood screening is visibly not a stand-alone strategy but, rather, an extra component to whatever form BTS take in a particular country. In practice, there may be substantial overlaps between CSW peer education projects and other HIV prevention strategies. If VCT is integrated with other services, the costing will need to keep in mind which activities should be excluded. These activities may comprise partner notification, assistance to support groups, preventive therapy for TB and treatment of STD.

Specifying Each Options

Once the question to be answered is known, the object of the costing and the scope of the work have been defined, and it is clear what alternatives are being costed, the exercise can proceed to describe each alternative in detail. For this, it is useful to be clear about how costs will be classified. To undertake cost analysis of HIV prevention, a primary classification by input and organisational level is suggested. It is also useful to make a secondary classification of the strategies by the activities that are taking place within them. This helps ascertain that costs are not duplicated or omitted between inputs and activities. It also provides a framework by which a strategy can be costed by activity if this is considered useful for decision-making.

Inputs

The most common inputs present across all strategies are listed in Table 1 as follows. While costing a particular project, it is necessary to give in detail the inputs within each category.

TABLE 1
CLASSIFICATION OF COSTS BY MAIN INPUT CATEGORIES

Capital Costs	*Recurrent Costs*
Buildings	Personnel
Equipment	Supplies
Vehicles	Vehicle operating and maintenance
Consultancies (non-recurrent)	Building operating and maintenance
	Consultancies (recurrent)
	Other (including media fees)

It is important to keep in mind that all items that have a life of more than a year are treated as capital items. Thus all IEC material, training and consultancies, whose effect is expected to last more than a year, should be treated as capital item. So as to gauge whether an item lasts for more than one year, it is important to look at the frequency of the item in the project - e.g. how often refresher training is provided.

Activities

Treating Activities as inputs: Another cost which may look like an input category is start-up activities. Although in reality this is an activity, adding activities to the input list can be logical in certain cases. "If one activity is clearly separate from the others, both financially and administratively, it may be easier not to attempt to break it down into its component physical inputs, but merely to record the total cost. For example, start-up, training and social mobilization activities are treated as categories of inputs and included alongwith personnel, vehicles and the like. When this is done, it is assumed that all the resources required for the activity (e.g. personnel and vehicles) are included in that category (e.g. training) and not under the separate categories of personnel, vehicles, and so forth. Thus, the full cost of all inputs used for training is estimated and used as the value for that category" (PHC:9). Start-up, training and social mobilization activities whose impact is expected to last more than one year are classified as capital items.

Consultancies are also regarded as an input. It is, therefore, important to ascertain that none of the consultancy costs are double-counted. For example, fees and allowances paid to individuals working on a consultancy input should not also be costed in the personnel inputs.

Resource inputs combine to achieve targets of the activities. It is useful to present cost data by activity. Bringing together measures of cost and output by 'activity' rather than by the more aggregated 'strategy' can provide an additional tool in project evaluation. Each HIV prevention strategy is likely to include a range of activities, some of which will be common across all strategies and some of which will be unique to particular strategies. Table 3 displays a classification of activity by strategy.

TABLE 2
CLASSIFICATION OF STRATEGIES BY ACTIVITY

Strategy	*Activities*
1. HIV blood screening	*Donor recruitment* - including everything related to motivating, educating, recruiting, selecting, screening, counselling and retaining blood donors.
	Blood Collection - including all costs of collecting blood from accepted donors.
	HIV testing - including the first and any subsequent confirmatory tests.
	Blood processing - including all costs (except HIV testing) related to the processing of blood, including other testing, blood grouping, preparation of blood products, and all measures taken to ensure safety of blood prior to storage.
	Blood storage/distribution - including all steps taken in storing and transporting blood through to its final transfusion in hospital.
	Training - training of all personnel, including laboratory, medical, managerial and support staff.
	Management and administration - including planning and supervision of the strategy.

Strategy	Activities
2. Mass Media	*Development and production of IEC materials* - often includes focus group discussions and market research; testing, revision and re-testing of messages with sample audiences; and translation of the materials into a range of local languages. The costs of the production of the IEC materials, once they are designed, should also be included here.
	Transmission/distribution of IEC materials and messages- modes and costs of transmission will vary according to the type of media being used. Sometimes these activities will include pre-publicity by advertising firms, for example prior to launching television or radio dramas.
	Management and administration - including costs of the overheads of the campaign, planning costs and the cost of evaluating the strategy (including baseline surveys and post-campaign evaluations).
3. HIV School education	*Development and production of curriculum and educational materials* - includes preliminary work such as focus group discussions and testing, revision and re-testing of messages with sample audiences, as well as the production of the final materials. There may also be continuous production of materials for the project, for example when an AIDS magazine or newsletter is established.
	Training - a variety of school staff may be taken away from their routine activities and given training to implement the new curriculum. Ideally, training should address teaching methods as well as provide information on AIDS. If the new curriculum becomes an on-going activity, staff should be given refresher training as well as initial training.
	Implementation of curriculum - comprises in-school teaching activities of the staff responsible for teaching the AIDS curriculum.
	Management/administration - day-to-day management and administration of the strategy by the

Strategy	Activities
	overseeing department (for example the Ministry of Education or Ministry of Health); also includes the costs of planning and evaluating the strategy.
4. Condom social marketing	*Development and production of IEC materials* - may include market research, testing, re-testing and any necessary translation. Although promotional materials may be produced for mass media transmission, some may also be produced for more local distribution, particularly in countries where explicit advertising of condoms is restricted. Local promotional materials may include such items as calendars, diaries, key rings, stickers and T-shirts. Technical assistance from specialist marketing consultants is commonly brought in from time to time during the project. *Training* - includes retailers receiving some guidance on the correct use of condoms so that they can relay this information, and possibly other HIV prevention information, to their customers. Necessary training may be undertaken by the social marketing organisation or contracted to the commercial manufacturer. *Transmission of IEC materials/messages* - includes all advertising and promotion activities. Activities may include sponsored conferences and professional seminars, award ceremonies for achievement, use of mass media, face-to-face distribution of promotional materials through health professionals, pharmacists, midwives, traditional birth attendants, traditional healers, shopkeepers and itinerant salesman, and mass distribution in hotels, bars and companies. *Condom distribution* - includes costs of storing and packaging the condoms as well as distributing them to wholesalers or retailers. Distribution channels may be private or public sector or both. Packaging and distributing may be contracted out. *Management and administration* - includes day-to-day activities, planning and evaluation activities

Strategy	Activities
	and technical support from management consultants.
5. STD treatment	*Development/distribution of diagnostic and treatment protocols* - this may include strengthening of existing laboratory facilities. *Training* - including clinical and support staff. *Diagnosis* - includes both laboratory and syndromic diagnosis. *Counselling* - including drug and condom provision. *Partner notification* - partner tracing, notification and counselling. *Management and administration* - including planning, supervision and evaluation.
6. Sex worker peer education	*Development and production of IEC materials* - for the target population. *Recruitment of peer educators* - can be thought of as a social mobilization component in the project. This activity will occur throughout the lifetime of the project, although the main recruitment will occur at the beginning. Both staff and other peer educators could do this. *Training* - of all staff and particularly of the CSW peer educators who will have responsibility for conducting the educational sessions; includes refresher training. *Transmission of IEC materials/messages* - to the target population, through individual and/or group sessions. *Condom distribution/sales.* *Management and administration* - including planning, supervision and evaluation of the strategy.
7. Voluntary counselling and testing	*Development and production of IEC materials* - clients may be shown a video, or handed educational materials at the pre-test counselling session; materials require development, testing, and production. *Training* - counsellors need to be trained in appropriate techniques, with fully-trained counsellors available to conduct the training and supervise staff with lesser levels of training.

Strategy	*Activities*
	Counselling pre-test - done with individuals, couples, or groups. Individual counselling may be followed or preceded by a group session, sometimes involving showing a video. Condoms may be distributed free of charge or sold. Blood may be drawn immediately for those who decide to proceed with the test, or at a separate visit.
	Testing - laboratory testing of blood may be done on site or at a central facility.
	Counselling post-test - all individuals may be given their results at a post-test counselling session, or only those found positive.
	Management and administration - especially for the free-standing centres, there will be a number of management activities to be carried out.
8. Harm reduction	*Development and production of IEC materials* - often includes focus group discussions and market research; testing, revision and re-testing of messages with sample audiences; and translation of the materials into a range of local languages. The costs of the production of the IEC materials once they are designed should also be included here.
	Transmission/distribution of IEC materials and messages-modes and costs of transmission will vary according to the type of media being used.
	Recruitment of peer educators - can be thought of as a social mobilization component in the project. This activity will occur throughout the lifetime of the project, although the main recruitment will occur at the beginning, Both staff and other peer educators could do this.
	Counselling - designed to decrease risky behaviour, such as sharing equipment.
	Syringe/Needle Exchange - exchange of used needles/ syringes for clean ones.
	Disposal of contaminated needles - this could include provision of sharp containers, transport, biohazard disposal and possible incineration.
	Bleaching/Distribution of substances to clean- equipment-distribution of, and advice on, cleaning solutions.

Strategy	Activities
	Condom distribution - includes costs of storing and packaging the condoms as well as distributing them to wholesalers or retailers.
	HIV testing - including the first and any subsequent confirmatory tests and counselling pre- and post-test.
	Referral to other services - includes referral to other medical services (e.g. STD treatment), social welfare and legal support.
	Training - training of all personnel, including laboratory, medical, managerial and support staff.
	Management and administration - including planning and supervision of the project.
9. Mother-to-child transmission	*Strengthening Antenatal facilities* - including provision for HIV testing.
	Training - of staff.
	Purchasing and storage of ARV drugs and replacement feeding.
	Counselling - before notification of results, during ARV regimen and for follow-up
	Management and administration - including planning and supervision of project and follow-up of mothers and infants.

In practice, not all stated activities may be happening within the implementation of a particular strategy. Nevertheless it is likely that implementation of each strategy involves some combination of these activities. In some cases, a resource input, as described in the primary classification, will be used solely for one activity and, in other cases, it will be shared between activities. For instance, in a government STD clinic, drug inputs may be entirely consumed by the 'STD treatment' activity, whilst a clinician's time may be divided between 'STD treatment', 'counselling', 'condom distribution' and 'management and administration'.

Observations of Activities: HIV Prevention Strategies

Some specific observations about activities in different HIV prevention strategies:

HIV Blood Screening: In a developed BTS, the majority of these activities will have been taking place before implementation of HIV blood screening, It might, therefore, be convenient to assume that an HIV screening strategy can be costed by measuring only the incremental costs of adding the HIV blood testing. The situation is, not as simple. In areas where HIV prevalence is high, replacement of discarded blood can entail the main cost of HIV safety. The cost of HIV blood screening can, therefore, depend more upon the costs incurred on pre-testing activities than on the costs of HIV testing itself. For this reason, it is not enough to measure only the incremental costs of the HIV blood testing activity. Rather, the costs of implementing an HIV blood screening strategy will include the costs of all resources used in undertaking the HIV testing, as well as the full replacement cost of the blood that tests HIV-positive and is discarded.

The unit costs of this blood will include the costs of donor recruitment, selection and counselling, blood collection, tests conducted before the HIV test, and a proportionate share of overheads such as administration and staff training, supervision and management. To find out such units costs, the costs of some activities will have to be obtained for the wider BTS and divided to the strategy activities in question. For instance, management and administration costs are likely to be shared between pre-testing and post-testing activities and laboratory costs may be shared between HIV tests and other tests. Having set out this far into a costing exercise, it might be relevant to obtain costs for the BTS as a whole, rather than go half way and measure only those costs connected to the HIV screening strategy. How to conduct a costing exercise will depend upon the objectives of that exercise and the audience interested in the results. The manager of a BTS may be wanting not only the cost of making blood HIV-safe but also more detailed and more generally applicable cost data. By costing the whole BTS, total costs can be presented by activity and the proportion of costs incurred by the HIV blood screening strategy can also be disaggregated. If a full costing is deemed appropriate, detailed guidance can be sought from WHO's Costing of Blood Transfusion Services.

CSW: There may be other complementary activities taking

place, like initiatives to access clients for educational sessions. Other activities for CSW projects may not be directly connected to HIV prevention, e.g. creche and income-support activities.

VCT: Some centres give support to HIV-positive groups, but this is not acknowledged as a core activity of a VCT service.

IDU: In reality, not all stated activities may be going on within the implementation of a particular strategy. Nevertheless it is possible that implementation of each strategy entails some combination of these activities. In some cases, a resource input, as given in the primary classification, will be used solely for one activity and, in other cases, it will be shared between activities. For instance a clinician's time may be divided between 'STD treatment', 'counselling', 'condom distribution' and management and administration'.

What to include if calculating costs in a clinical trial

Very often cost and cost-effectiveness analyses of HIV prevention strategies are carried out in the context of on-going clinical trials. In order to consider the feasibility of delivering these services, it is necessary to include all costs that were necessary to ensure the functioning of the project. For instance, if the project had to provide additional basic infrastructure before looking at the success of a particular intervention, the costs of this basic infrastructure should be included. Similarly, it is necessary to exclude costs associated with the research dimension of the intervention (e.g. some components of monitoring and evaluation).

Organisational Level

Some of the HIV prevention strategies may consist of activities at a number of organisational levels. National programmes may operate from the field in districts and regions up to central-level administration. While moving up organisational levels in the hierarchy, away from the point of service delivery, it can become more and more difficult to get data and to take out relevant costs. Which costs at each organisational level are to be included in the costing study will depend upon the amount of responsibility of the decision-maker who is supposed to use the results, and the way in which the results will be applied. It is suggested that a full costing be conducted at the main service delivery level. For higher organisational levels, it is suggested that personnel inputs be costed, and that any other additional or incremental costs incurred by adding the HIV prevention strategy to existing work.

Where HIV prevention is combined with other work, the incremental cost of its addition may be very negligible at regional and national levels. Using this approach means that the main inputs to be costed at the higher organisational levels are personnel, vehicle use and, supplies. Overheads at those organisational levels, like buildings, office equipment, utilities and general administration, can generally be excluded. Where, however, new HIV prevention strategies need substantial new administrative, logistic or technical support from more central levels, these incremental costs will require a wider range of inputs and be more substantial.

These inputs should be costed and appropriately allocated to the AIDS strategy. For instance, the cost of strengthening the National AIDS Control Programme to support a new preventive strategy should be costed in that strategy. In order to find out the organisational level, it is necessary to consider the range of service providers available for a project or programme. Again, these will vary by strategy:

HIV blood screening: The more localized the costing study, the more it is possible that it will be concerned with just one provider. On the other hand, a national strategy may include a number of providers. For instance, in Zaire the mining industry is responsible for a substantial proportion of transfusions but transfusions are also available in the public and private sectors. Which providers to include should be determined from the objectives of the study and, specially, from consideration of the decision-making audience. Decisions about the organisational levels from which costs should be ascertained are likely to be considered from the objectives of each particular costing exercise.

If the BTS to be costed is localized - for example, HIV blood screening at one mission hospital - it may be important to cost only one service delivery level. If the study is focusing on national costs, it will probably have to consider costs at all organisational levels from the centre to the periphery. Starting from the centre and moving down through the system, cost information for each organisational level should be collected from expenditure records. If such expenditure records are not available, costs may need to be constructed from quantity and unit cost information collected during field visits. Fieldwork may need to be restricted to costing a representative sample of facilities at each of the organisational levels.

Mass media: At a given time, there may be many AIDS media campaigns being conducted in a country by both government and nongovernmental organisations. More so than in some of the other strategies, there can be a number of providers involved in the strategy, or even in one campaign. For instance, a radio drama in Zambia had the involvement of the Health Education Unit of the Ministry of Health, the Government National AIDS Prevention and Control Programme, the National Radio Corporation, a number of colleges and NGOs, drama groups, and the USAID public health communication support programme, AIDSCOM. A variety of Implementers an organisations will need to be examined for cost information. Some activities may be contracted out to commercial enterprises, for example IEC production to professional advertising agencies. This may make cost collection easy as the fees charged are likely to comprise of the agency's own overheads and support costs for the work carried out. In this case, the expenditure for the activity in question can be considered as an aggregate input rather than broken down into its constituent inputs.

A mass media campaign is generally implemented at the national level and activities are centralized. Costs may, therefore, need to be collected from only one organisational level although there may be a number of providers involved at that level. Costs obtained will be those directly spent by a particular campaign plus an adequate share of the overhead costs of the organisation with primary responsibility for supervising, managing and administering the campaign or strategy. This could, for instance, be a share of the running costs of the Health Education Unit of a Ministry of Health or its equivalent. It is suggested that, apart from the lead agency in the campaign, no attempts be made to cost the overheads of other organisations with partial involvement in the strategy. A share of the personnel costs of those organisations should, however, be included, and distributed according to the share of staff time spent on the mass media campaign.

HIV school education: The main provider of this strategy is likely to be a government ministry, such as the Ministry of Education or Ministry of Health. Curriculum development and material production may be carried out by them or contracted out to a specialized agency. Similarly, training of staff may be undertaken by the Ministry or by a contracted agency. The actual teaching of AIDS education is done by staff in the schools included in the strategy. Donors may also give inputs to the strategy, for instance consultancies during the start-up phase. If the project is a more localized NGO initiative, the only providers involved may be the NGO and the schools in which they are implementing the strategy. Most of the costing data should be obtained centrally from the organisation with overall responsibility for the strategy - for instance, the relevant Ministry.

Costs of the time that school staff spend on the strategy during training and teaching may need to be collected from a sample of schools involved in the strategy. If any donors provide aid to the project, for example start-up technical aid, it may be necessary to approach them directly for details of the costs of their inputs. If the project is a more localized NGO initiative, cost data should be obtained directly from the NGO, and other costs, including personnel, from the schools in which the strategy is being implemented.

Condom social marketing: Several institutions are usually involved in a social marketing project. A foreign donor may provide consultancies in the start-up phase and on-going financial assistance. Either the donor or a commercial manufacturer could be the source of condoms. Within the country, most activities tend to be coordinated by a social marketing organisation. They may hire other organisations for marketing promotion, and distribution. The Ministry of Health or Family Welfare may participate in project policy, monitoring and distribution of the condoms through its own outlets. At the periphery, individual retailers will be buying and selling the condoms. In most cases, the social marketing organisation will have central expenditure records that collate the financial costs of these decentralized activities. To get the economic costs of the strategy, it may be necessary to deal with some of the other agencies directly. For instance, the social marketing organisation may not have information on the costs of donor inputs. Because of the social marketing organisation's role in centralizing expenditure data from decentralized project activities, the majority of costing information can be collected from that organisation's office. Field visits may, however, be necessary to collect extra data, for instance costs of any inputs that do not entail project expenditure. It may be necessary to contact the organisation's headquarters overseas as well as foreign donors for details of the costs of external inputs - for example, condoms and consultancies. Only direct contributions to the project should be included; overheads that are not included in the country project can be excluded.

Gathering Data from CSM Organisations

Key information to collect from the social marketing organisation includes the total cost of the project (and an idea of the methods used to calculate this figure); the number of condoms sold; project expenditure on condoms; and revenue giving to the project from condom sales. Social marketing organisations are usually instructed to share information, but it may be in their own format, which is not ideal for cost analysis. It may, therefore, be important to adapt such information as is available.

STD treatment: Any primary-level STD treatment service is may be provided by a single organisation, which could be a government, private for profit or NGO provider. At times, however, private or NGO facilities may receive government support for supervision, training or drug supplies. Some private and NGO facilities without their own laboratory or referral services may depend on government facilities for these.

Government: If the study is considering national costs, it should look at costs at all levels from the centre to the periphery. Starting at the centre, cost information for levels below should be collected from expenditure records. If such expenditure records are not available, costs will need to be constructed from information collected through field visits to the lower levels. A sample of representative primary-level facilities should be included in the costing study. The costs of laboratory and referral services should also be added in the costing study and these may be incurred at higher organisational levels. Overhead and support costs for managing and administering the service may need to be gathered at a number of levels. In vertical systems, relevant costs at the different levels are likely to be well defined and should be included in their entirety. There may, for instance, be specific STD project offices at the national and provincial levels. Where STD services are combined horizontally with other services, it will be harder to calculate the costs that relate to support of the STD services. In this situation, only the incremental costs incurred in supporting the strategy should be taken, together with the costs of the time that personnel spend working on the strategy.

Private-for-profit and NGOs: Some projects may comprise of only one specialized STD clinic or one general clinic that gives STD treatment, and the costs for these may be collected from a visit to only one organisational level. In other cases the primary STD service may be attached to a private/NGO referral hospital and two organisational levels may have to be visited to obtain the necessary costing data.

Sex worker peer education: This type of approach is normally implemented by NGOs. A lead NGO may coordinate support from other NGOs as well as from national or international donors. At times, government institutions may provide some inputs to the project, such as condom supplies, building space or salary support. Donors may also provide condoms, as well as technical aid. Condoms may also be sold by peer educators rather than just distributed free. It may be important to deal with only one or two organisational levels to cost this kind of project. The main provider of data will be the NGO's management office. The second organisational level, for information that the NGO office is notable to provide, is the community level where peer educators carry out the educational activities, although at this level, the organisation may be much more informal. Government contributions may need to be examined separately, for instance at the district or municipal level. It may also be necessary to contact donors for the costs of their inputs.

VCT: Where VCT is provided by an array of agencies, the purpose of the study will determine whether a representative sample is required, or a study of the service thought to be most replicable or most successful. Where VCT centres are provided regularly by governments, and if the research looks at costs nationwide, costs will have to be collected at all levels from the centre to the periphery. Starting from the centre, cost information for levels below should be gathered from expenditure records. If these are not available, costs will need to be constructed through visits to lower levels. A sample of VCT facilities should be chosen for detailed costing. The incremental costs of support given to the VCT clinics by higher levels should be included.

If a VCT service provided by an NGO is being costed, there could be only one level of interest or, at most, the level of the service plus the incremental costs of support given from a head office. Since VCT services may be financed from a number of different sources, including NGOs, government subsidies, and external donors, a variety of funders may need to be approached at different levels to collect comprehensive cost data.

IDU: An IDU project is mostly implemented by NGOs. A lead NGO may coordinate support from other NGOs and from national or international donors. At times government institutions may give some inputs to the Project, such as condom supplies, building space or salary support. Donors may also provide condoms, as well as technical aid. Condoms may also be sold by peer educators rather than just distributed free.

Deciding on the Data Timeframe

In practice one should attempt to measure the costs incurred over one full year. This is likely to be in line with the records of most types of relevant data, such as expenditure on personnel and services provided. A one-year period prevents any distortions that may be caused by seasonal effects. At times, limitations of information, e.g., for a new programme, or for study time, might make it mandatory to choose a shorter period. If you study costs for less than one year, you might need to discuss with other knowledgeable persons ways of avoiding serious misrepresentations. It is thus suggested that, to increase accuracy and relevance of cost data, you should select the most recent year for which cost data are likely to be available. If the year chosen is too much in the past, important information may be lost. If the year is too recent, some routinely collected statistics may not yet be available. All times the financial year is not the same as the calendar year. If this is the case, possibilities should be worked out to obtain disaggregated data for each month covering costs or effectiveness, so that you can build up either annual effectiveness data for the financial year or expenditure figures for the calendar year. If you are collecting more than one year's worth of information, then you need to keep proper track of which year the expenditure took place.

While undertaking a costing exercise, cost data can be gathered retrospectively from such sources as accounting records, questionnaires and interviews. Information systems can also be specially established to collect costing data prospectively over a suitable time period. Once collected, these data will also be examined retrospectively. Costs may vary during the course of a project's implementation, especially if there are high initial start-up costs. These costs are connected with start-up activities that are conducted at the beginning of a project and rarely repeated, such as buying of vehicles or project infrastructure. For instance, development of standard diagnostic protocols may be one of the start-up costs of an STD treatment strategy. If start-up costs are being included in the costing, they should be calculated in the same way as capital costs and annualized over the expected lifetime of the project.

Varying timeframes for data collection may be chosen depending upon the objectives of costing studies, in particular. Emphasis on types of costs may vary depending upon the type of situation:

(i) Focus on operational efficiency and modification of on-going projects may require that start-up costs may be ignored and only on-going recurrent and annualized capital costs collected. If only on-going costs of routine services are being considered, it is suggested that annual costs be collected for a recent appropriate year. They should include recurrent costs and annualized capital costs.

(ii) If the study is seeking data on total project costs, costs should be recorded for all years in which they were incurred. These costs will comprise start-up costs such as planning, staff recruitment and project site identification.

(iii) Identification. This is particularly necessary for CSM, as unit costs tend to decrease over the life of a CSM project due to the increasing volume of sales. While making comparisons between projects, it is necessary to keep in mind how long each project has been going on. CSM projects tend to have high start-up costs incurred in market research, project design and project launch.

(iv) If the costing exercise relates to future modification or sustainability of the project, the costs of on-going activities (including depreciation of capital inputs) should be collected from a regular phase of the project. These should necessarily be costs for the most recent year for which data are available. If costs are collected from a period early in the project, it is important to exclude one-off start-up costs that would inflate estimates of the resources required to run the project in the future.

(v) If information is needed on the costs of replicating the project, all costs incurred over the span of the project since its inception should be collected. This comprises both start-up and on-going activities. Costs incurred in all years of the project should be recorded, including the costs of organisational changes made as part of the HIV prevention strategy. For instance, for HIV blood screening, changes may comprise establishing a national BTS for the first time, revamping an already established BTS, adding facilities such as laboratories, or adding a new set of tests in laboratories. Start-up costs may also comprise of operations such as the establishment of new national policies for BTS blood-screening practice.

(vi) The chosen timeframe may also depend on the maturation of the project. If the approach is of limited duration, a costing exercise may need to cover all costs, including those incurred by start-up activities. If the strategy has become institutionalized and is now an established operation, it may be relevant for the costing exercise to investigate on-going costs only.

Mass media: campaigns will normally be a time-bound discontinuous exercise rather than a continuous on-going set of activities. Due to this, each mass media campaign is most appropriately costed from its conception to completion. The costing exercise will, thus include all costs rather than differentiate between start-up and on-going costs in the way appropriate for some of the other strategies. If the objective is to cost a broader strategy that is, in fact, on-going, the strategy as a whole may comprise a series of campaigns. It may then be necessary to cost overheads for developing and overseeing the series, alongwith costing each campaign.

To carryout cost-effectiveness analysis it is necessary that data on both costs and effectiveness be connected in such a way that only the costs of those resources that produce the effects are included. It is usually a suggested practice to calculate both costs and effects over the period of a year. Nonetheless, consideration needs to be made regarding what is most suitable for a particular strategy. One year of cost data may be appropriate for prevention activities that are on-going, for instance blood screening programmes. However, in some strategies, such as mass media campaigns, costs may be incurred over a shorter span of time whereas effects may be fact over a longer time period in the future. In all cases, it is necessary that a record be made of the timeframe to which data refer. If cost data have been gathered from more than one year, it will be necessary to convert them to a constant Base Year value before adding them together. The selected Base Year should ideally be the most recent year for which data are available.

Selecting a Sample

At times it may be necessary to cost a national programme which includes geographically, dispersed and multiple units, for instance a national blood transfusion service or STD programme. In this case, it may be appropriate to cost-only a sample of facilities from each organisational level or levels. Even while costing a more localized project such as a peer education project, it may be important to sample time allocations of representative members of staff during representative weeks of the year.

There are many ways in which you can choose. Usually, in taking a sample, you are not just interested in the particular units you select. You may need to draw conclusions about the population as a whole whereby, there are certain rules you must follow. Statisticians have devised many different ways to satisfy the conditions necessary to allow valid conclusions to be drawn about the population from samples. Four of these methods are described below. For each of them, the size of the sample drawn will influence the degree to which the statistical variation will affect the reliability in the estimate for the whole population. Disregarding expense and other problems, the larger the sample, the more the confidence. Another factor is the extent of variation among units of the population; smaller variations allow a smaller sample size. You might wish to consult a statistician about these matters. One of the standard approaches to selection is random sampling. This is a good method to use if you can feasibly list (and number) all the elements of the entire population and if there are no subgroups you are specifically interested in. You could, for example, use it in choosing health centres within a district. Having chosen the sample size, you would select the required number of units at random from a numbered list, using a table of random numbers.

Systematic sampling is a second approach. It is simpler to use than simple random sampling, and is most useful when there are large numbers in the population (say, patients attending a hospital). The procedure is as follows:

(a) Get a list of units (n) (in no systematic order) from which the sample is to be chosen.
(b) Decide on the size of the sample (s).
(c) Calculate the ratio n/s (=k). Select every kth item on the list, starting at any point. For example, if you want a sample of 50 patients (i.e. s = 50) out of 2000 attending the clinic in a year (i.e. n = 2000). Then k = 2000/50 = 40, and you would then select every 40th patient. If s does not divide exactly into n, e.g. k = 40.54, then round k up or down to the nearest whole number.

If you were interested in the health centre costs of a PHC programme in the country as a whole, studying a random (or stratified) sample would probably require a lot of travelling and effort, since these units are likely to be widespread.

An alternative approach is to first choose a sample of districts and then to look at the health centre costs only in those districts.

This is called cluster sampling. It gives less reliable results than pure random sampling, but can have major logistical advantages. First, choose a random sample to determine the clusters (in this case, districts) to be studied; then, in the selected clusters, either choose all the units (health centres) or a random sample of them.

A fourth approach with a formal statistical basis is stratified sampling. You may be interested in ensuring that you include units with particular characteristics in your sample (e.g. health centres in both rural and urban areas), so that you can compare them. For this, first divide the total population (in this case, all the health centres) into subgroups (urban and rural); then take a random or systematic sample or even a clustered sample in each subgroup.

Even though the mathematical advantages of the above approaches are well known to specialists, there are situations when a less formal, but more practical, sampling technique might be selected, which may be referred to as judgement sampling. In a significant number of practical cases, barriers to statistical sampling might exist, for instance, excessive costs or limited co-operation from staff in specific delivery units. When one of these problems takes place, random sampling may not be possible, and you may require to use your own judgement to select a reasonably typical group of units for study. The practical advantages of this method are evident, but the inability to draw general conclusions about the entire population on a formal statistical basis is a clear limitation the use of a judgement sample. It is considered a less than ideal, but occasionally practical, approach to the task of choosing the sample. The basis upon which any sample is selected should be clearly reported in the presentation of results. When the costs of the sample facilities or activities are examined, it will be important to multiply these data up to acquire costs for the population that the sample represented.

Work Schedule

Three important ground rules in the process of data collection are:

(i) Collect the information at the highest organisational level at which it is available for main service delivery (if it is of reasonable quality) to reduce study time and expense.

(ii) Avoid counting the same cost element (input) twice ('double counting') when you have collected data at more than one level (for instance, when staffing or salary figures have been provided at both the delivery-unit and higher levels).

(iii) Put your greatest endeavour into finding (and using) information on the largest input categories rather than the smaller, less important categories (such as supplies and building operation in most programmes). The latter can often be collected by rough calculations, perhaps based on rules of thumb, such as assuming operating costs of buildings to be equal to a certain percentage of their annual capital costs.

Ten

Collection and Analysis of Cost Data

Instructions about how to collect cost data and make relevant adjustments to the data to suit the need of the cost analysis are very important for the proper implementation of the cost analysis.

Financial and Economic Costs

It is essential to know the difference between financial and economic costs before learning how to collect data, as in some cases it will be important to carry out analysis with one rather than the other. By having different columns for financial and economic costs, the worksheets record clearly which inputs comprise actual project expenditure (financial costs) and which are attributed to economic costs. If the costing exercise is conducted to undertake a cost-effectiveness analysis, then all resources consumed should be valued in terms of their opportunity cost, i.e. their full economic cost.

Differences

There are three main ways in which economic costs are different from financial costs:

Donated items: The economic cost or value of donated goods and services can most easily be calculated by taking their equivalent market prices. For instance, in the case of radio time you could find out what the radio station normally charges for advertising, keeping in mind the duration and time of day. In case of volunteer labour, you could investigate whether those people receive a salary or wages elsewhere and use that for costing their donated time. Varying degrees of effort can be put into deriving economic costs. Donated goods and services should always be valued.

In cases where input price is wrong or distorted: If some of the consumed resources have market prices that do not reflect their true value - for example they are too low due to subsidies, too high because of inclusion of transfer taxes or are distorted through government-set foreign exchange rates - it may be necessary to replace the stated prices with 'shadow prices' for purposes of analysis. "Economists use the term 'shadow price' to refer to a price that has been adjusted for various reasons, including donations, to yield economic cost" (PHC: 58). The actual shadow price you use will depend on the nature of the good. For instance, if official exchange rates are distorted, you may want to use prevailing black market rates.

It is suggested that an attempt be made on shadow pricing in proportion to the contribution that the resource in question makes to the total cost of the project.

Capital goods: are defined as inputs that last for more than one year. If you studied expenditure only for one particular year, you may get a distorted view of long-term average annual costs. For instance, a great deal of equipment might have been purchased in the year earlier, with no expenditure on capital at all during the study period. One way to identify long-term financial commitments is annualize or spread out costs by:

(a) identify all the capital goods being used in that year;
(b) find out the current (replacement) cost of purchasing them (C);
(c) estimate the total years each is likely to last from when it was purchased (N) (the 'working life' or 'useful life');
(d) estimate the average annual cost of each capital item in terms of a simple 'straight line' depreciation. (PHC: 32-33).

This average annual cost is what you would require for the cost of each capital item for one year under financial costs.

"With economic costs, you will usually be concerned with the cost of resources used over a specific period (say, one year), rather than at the time they are purchased. Simply obtaining the straight-line of capital items is a way of spreading capital costs over a period of time, but it is not adequate if one is interested in economic costs, which must take into account the value of alternative opportunities for using the resources tied up in the capital inputs.

"To calculate the economic cost of capital on an 'annualized' (cost per year) basis, use the following approach.

(a) *Current value.* Estimate the current value of the capital item, as the amount you would have to pay to purchase a similar item now (i.e. the replacement value rather than the original price).

(b) *Useful life.* Estimate the total number of years of useful life the item can realistically be expected to have (from the time of purchase).

(c) *Discount rate.* Find out the discount rate used by the economic planning office or Ministry of Finance. Annualisation factor. Consult a standard table (found at the end of this chapter) to find the correct annualization factor.

(d) *Calculation of annual cost.* Calculate the annual cost by dividing the current value of the item by the annualization factor. This factor is determined by the discount rate and useful life of the item.

"For a single $10,000 piece of equipment with a useful life of 5 years, the approach above would be applied as follows:

- Discount rate: 10 per cent.
- Annualizing factor (from standard table)- 3.791.
- Calculation of annual economic cost- $10,000/3.791 = $2,638 per year (rounded figure).

"To compare this economic cost with the corresponding financial cost, note that the latter would be $10,000/5 = $2,000 per year. The investment of funds 'up front', to pay for the equipment in full at the start of its use, raises the annual economic cost - which is to be expected" (PHC- 59-61).

The practical steps to be taken in collecting are very similar whether financial or economic cost data. Each worksheet in the Annex is designed in such a way that financial and economic costs can be clearly distinguished and it is important that the two categories of cost are not mixed up. Whether economic or financial costs are used, whether a manager analysing financial costs prefers to take a project budget perspective and exclude costs of donated goods, or to take a wider perspective and include them, and whether or not shadow pricing is introduced into economic costs, will be dependant on the objectives of the costing study being undertaken. The worksheets are designed keeping in mind these different purposes. It is always important to accurately record the way in which economic costs have been obtained from financial costs.

Collecting Background Data

The information recorded on the background data sheet is required for analysis of the cost data, including calculation of economic costs, where needed, and for making the results of the study more conclusive. The informational needed can usually be collected from the Central Economic Planning Office, the Finance Ministry or the Central Bank. Which of these is more accessible may, in practice, be based upon contacts between the officials with whom one is dealing in the health or other ministries, and in these other institutions. The numbers noted should be the average figures for the Base Year. The choice of discount rate-a rate that reflects the opportunity cost of tying up funds in the project-is particularly important as it can significantly influence the relative cost-effectiveness of strategies being compared. If there is no particular suggested rate for the country, then a rate can be taken from economic project appraisals done by other organisations such as the World Bank. A more difficult approach would be to calculate the real rate of interest, i.e. the rate of interest that would be attained by depositing the money in the bank minus the rate of interest. Alternatively, an easier approach is to take a 'high side' World Bank discount rate of 10 per cent. The effects of using different rates can be seen by conducting sensitivity analyses. In order to see how sensitive your results are to the choice of rate, you can visualize three scenarios: (a) your choice of rate; (b) twice that rate; and (c) half that rate. Then the costs should be calculated based on these three different scenarios, so as to determine if your analysis is highly sensitive to your assumptions.

Gathering the Input Data (Form C)

The main tool for data collection in the field is through this set of forms. A set of 'C' forms can be collated for each organisational level (see discussion in previous chapter) if data are being recorded manually, each set should be stapled together and attached to a Form 'B' summary sheet, by organisational level. The Form C consists of separate forms under it for each category of input as follows:

C1 - capital costs: buildings
C2 - capital costs: equipment
C3 - capital costs: vehicles
C4 - capital costs: consultancies
C5a - recurrent costs: personnel
C5b - example of personnel time allocation form
C6 - recurrent costs: supplies
C7 - recurrent costs: vehicles operation and maintenance
C8 - recurrent costs: building operation and maintenance
C9 - recurrent costs: consultancies
C10 - recurrent costs: other

Best estimates often have to be made for some costs for which there is not much surety. If these costs represent a substantial proportion of the overall total, the effects of changing the estimates can be explored by doing sensitivity analyses same as the method used on discount rates above.

Gathering Data at the Different Organisational Levels: The B Forms

The 'B' forms have been made so as to accommodate collation of costs in as many organisational levels are adequate to the costing exercise in hand. The number of levels included is likely to differ according to the strategy, the type of service provider and the questions being addressed. The 'B' forms can themselves then be collated and totalled into a single Form 'A', which is a cost summary sheet for the strategy.

Currency

Forms should generally be filled and worked in the local currency and this currency should be mentioned on all forms. Where inputs have been bought in foreign currency, you will need to differentiate between those purchased from inside the country, and those purchased from abroad.

Where an input, such as office rent, has been bought in foreign currency inside the country, the amount should be converted to the equivalent price in local currency. For this, use the market exchange rate at the time the cost was incurred. The foreign exchange price should also be stated in a footnote on the form.

Where an input has been purchased in foreign currency from abroad, convert its cost to Base Year costs first, and then convert this figure into local currency using the market exchange rate for the Base Year (see 'Converting to constant prices ahead'). When an organisation maintains all its records in US dollars, it is recommended that conversion to local currency take place at the end of the costing exercise.

Source of Funds

All 'C' forms consist of a column in which to note the source of funds for each input. Information on source of funds may be specially important for planning the sustainability of programmes and for calculating the cost to private individuals for the prevention services that they receive. Funding sources are likely to include:

(i) Ministry of Health (all organisational levels)
(ii) Other ministry (specify)
(iii) Municipality/local authority
(iv) NGO/community groups
(v) Private for-profit organisation
(vi) Private individual
(vii) External donor (specify)

It is suggested that a list of funders be drawn up for each project and that each main source of funds be given a code to simplify data entry on the forms.

Source of Data

Each form also has a column to record the source of cost data by input. The source of data stated should consist of both the organisational source, for example, Accounts Department in the Ministry of Health, and the type of source, for instance balance sheets, interviews, accounting records or questionnaires.

Converting of Costs to Constant Prices

If cost data have been gathered from more than one year it will be necessary to convert them to a constant Base Year value before adding years together. This is due to the fact that inflation causes the value of money to change from one year to another. When it comes to data analysis, the most recent year for which data were available should be chosen as the Base Year and costs in all other years should be converted to their equivalent values in the Base Year. For instance, if costing data were collected from 1990 to 1999, then 1999 should be taken as the Base Year. This conversion is made using measures of domestic inflation such as Consumer Price Indices that should be obtained from the Finance Ministry, National Bank or Department of Statistics.

To convert expenditure in year Y to the prices of the chosen Base Year, multiply the expenditure in year Y by the consumer price index for the Base Year and divide by the consumer price index for year Y. If foreign exchange has been used to purchase inputs from inside the country, it is desirable still to use the domestic price index. However, if foreign currency has been used to purchase inputs from abroad, then a suitable foreign price index should be used to convert the sum to constant prices. For instance, if a vehicle is bought with US$ from the United States in 1990, then in order to convert prices to the Base Year 1999, a US Price Index must be used for that vehicle cost. First convert 1990 $ to 1999 (Base Year) $ and then convert into local currency for 1994, using 1994 market exchange rates. The bottom row of the final two columns of each Form 'C' should be used to convert the total financial or economic costs into total costs for the Base Year.

Suggestions on Importance of noting down time: Generally data are available for a number of years. It is necessary to be consistent in terms of the time frame that you use for the cost analysis. If you are gathering data from different years, it is important to mention this variable by variable. It is helpful to have a separate set of sheets C1-C10, with each set corresponding to one year. The importance of noting down the year is felt as you try to convert exchange rates (you need to use the exchange rate that is suitable for the time-period).

If you are collecting from different time-periods and want total costs for the entire period, you need to convert the data to the same year, using the domestic inflation rate.

Collecting of Data

Capital Resources

Capital resources are those resources that have a life expectancy of more than one year.

(a) Buildings (Form C1)

Buildings comprise health centres, hospitals, offices, staff houses and warehouses.

Financial cost: We suggest costing the buildings being used for implementation of the strategy by noting the annual rent (if rented) or by estimating the equivalent annual rent (if owned).

> "This means obtaining an estimate of the annual price charged for renting similar space. The estimate should distinguish between furnished and unfurnished buildings and between air-conditioned and non-air-conditioned space. In effect, this approach treats buildings as recurrent, instead of capital, inputs. You will probably need the assistance of a real-estate agent or someone else who is familiar with the rental market in the area" (PHC: 52).

Each building being used should be noted in column 1 of Form C1 and the source of funds for the building given in column 2. The actual annual rent or equivalent rent for a similar unfurnished building should be noted in column 3. Ten per cent of the annual rent price should be noted in column 5 to cover the costs of furnishings. The total of these two costs may then be noted in column 6. There may also be field offices located in other cities, whose costs should also be taken into account.

If there are buildings that are only rented occasionally for implementation of the strategy, the actual rent over the course of a year should be recorded in column 6. It is assumed that any space rented for such short-term use is furnished and that it is, thus not required to add extra costs for furnishings.

Economic Cost: Use of some premises may be made free of cost. For instance, the Ministry of Health may reserve a room in the Ministry to oversee the strategy. Although this involves no financial cost to the project itself, the provision of such premises does comprise economic opportunity cost. An economic analysis should value that space in case free provision is not possible in the future; for instance, if the space is used by another project. The cost at market rates to hire or rent such space, as and when it is requested, over the course of a year should be noted in column 4. However, it is possible that, if an organisation had to give rent, it would choose to move to a different, cheaper, area. It may be required to make a couple of estimates of opportunity cost, e.g. rent in city centre as well as rent out-of-town. An attempt need not be made to cost the capital overheads of other organisations with partial involvement in the strategy. Any agency to which work is contracted out is, in any case, expected to include a proportionate share of its overheads - including buildings - in its fees.

Suggestions regarding floor space: If you are trying to obtain an annual rent for a space, It is useful to know the floor space (e.g. in square metres or square feet). Commercial rents are often quoted in terms of this floor space. If the area is unknown, you may want to do a rough approximation by pacing out the length and width of space.

Allocation: If buildings are shared, a proportion of their costs should be apportioned to HIV/AIDS prevention according to floor space used, or as a percentage of total floor space for which rent is being quoted and/or by the share of time that that space is used for the AIDS work. The allocated percentage and the resulting cost should be entered in columns 8 and/or 9.

Strategy-specific Comments

(i) HIV blood screening is like to have incremental resource effect only if laboratories are newly made or if reorganisation of the system to accommodate the HIV prevention 'strategy necessitates new buildings.

(ii) implementing HIV school education may not need any additional space in schools. Capital costs of the schools can, therefore, be excluded. Only capital costs of lead agencies such as the Ministry of Education should be taken into account.

(iii) Capital costs tend to be a small part of overall project costs including social marketing projects, sex worker peer education projects and HIV prevention projects among IDU users.

(iv) In vertical systems, where premises are used only for STD or VCT services, the capital and recurrent costs of buildings should be attributed to the strategy. For STD or VCT services combined with other services at the primary level, and for joint laboratory facilities, the capital and recurrent costs of the buildings should be attributed to the strategy in proportion. These should be according to the space and/or time and/or activity indicators. At organisational levels above the primary level, only incremental costs of buildings need be costed against these strategies.

(b) Equipment (Form C2)

Capital equipment consist of supplies that are used for more than one year. Use the current cost for a similar piece of equipment, not the original purchase price. The cost should include freight. Sources of cost data could comprise recent government contracts, supply records from donors or local dealer estimates. The working life of a piece of equipment can be found out by asking individuals who operate it how long this type of equipment generally lasts before it is beyond repair (PHC: 33-34).

A useful method is to classify all capital equipment according to a unit price of $100 or more (unless national accounting procedures specify a different cut-off point) and these items should be listed in column 1 of Form C2, and the funding source for the equipment listed in column 2. Equipment with a unit price of less than $100 should be considered as a recurrent input and the cost noted on Form C6.

Financial Cost: The replacement price of the equipment should be listed in column 3. If the equipment is imported the foreign exchange price, consisting of freight and insurance, should be listed in column 3 and converted (see sections on 'Currency' and 'Converting to constant prices' in this chapter. The life expectancy or working life of the equipment when new should be listed in column 5. When such an estimate cannot be found, a five-year life can be standardized for most equipment. The average annual financial cost should be calculated by straight-line depreciation and entered in column 6.

Equipment, like audiovisual equipment, may need to be

bought for the development of the IEC materials. If the equipment will continue to be used throughout its life, then a proportion of its annualized costs should be attributed to the strategy or campaign being costed. If the equipment does not have any further use at the end of the project, its capital cost should be annualized over either its own life expectancy, or the length of the project, whichever is less. For instance, if the campaign is implemented from beginning to end in eight months, then two-thirds of the annualized cost of any equipment used exclusively for the strategy should be approached to the campaign. If, however, equipment purchased to produce the campaign has no foreseeable future use, the total capital costs of that equipment should be written off against the eight months period. It is assumed that the depreciation and running costs of equipment used by contracted organisations are included in their fees.

Economic cost: If the market replacement price is significantly different from the economic value of the equipment, a shadow price can be estimated and listed in column 4. This might be the case where equipment is imported and there is a wrong foreign exchange rate. The average annual economic cost of equipment can be calculated following the above methodology and entered in column 7.

Allocation: If equipment is shared between the HIV prevention strategy and other work as, for instance, National Blood Service laboratory equipment, costs should be apportioned according to the share of a relevant activity measure or by the proportion of time that the equipment is used for each. The allocated percentage and the resulting costs should be listed in columns 8 and/or 9.

Strategy-specific Comments

(i) An HIV blood-screening strategy is likely to include the purchase of new equipment if laboratory services are to be part of the strategy. These costs may be a substantial part of the total costs of the strategy.

(ii) For HIV education in schools, there will be only a limited requirement for equipment to implement the strategy.

(iii) A share of the equipment in the social marketing organisation's office should be apportioned to the strategy.

Such equipment as is required by the strategy will tend to be for the production of the promotion and marketing materials.

(iv) The majority of the equipment required for STD treatment is laboratory equipment but some diagnostic equipment will also be present in clinics. In specialized STD clinics, the full cost of this equipment should be added and, in integrated clinics, a share of the costs. The cost of the STD-related equipment should be allocated to the strategy according to the staff time allocations or by activity levels such as the percentage of total tests conducted that are for STD.

(v) For CSW peer education projects, the main requirement for equipment will be for training and education activities. Items like video cameras, televisions, video players, slide projectors, overhead projectors and computers may be bought specifically for the project.

(vi) For VCT, if the tests are carried out on the premises, then the separate elements of the costs of the tests need to be including the equipment. If the tests are done outside and charged for, then the fee can be taken as the financial cost of the test. If there is cause to believe that this cost is highly subsidized, then the test will need to be costed. If the test is free (for instance, done at a government hospital), then the actual cost of the test will require to be studied. The simplest method to cost the test will be to estimate the annual cost of the testing equipment and relevant laboratory staff and express the cost per HIV test done in a year.

(c) Vehicles (Form C3)

The kinds of vehicles you may require to value comprise bicycles, motorcycles, four-wheel-drive vehicles, cars and trucks. Use the current cost for a similar vehicle, not the original purchase price. The cost must include freight. Recent government contracts, supply records from donors, or local dealer estimates are handy sources of information. The working life of a vehicle will differ considerably, depending on type of vehicle, terrain, use and maintenance. For this you should try to obtain a local consensus on the expected working life of each type of vehicle. Question several people who use, drive or service cars for an estimate of the duration this type of vehicle has lasted in the past (i.e. how long before the vehicle reached a stage where it was not worth repairing). For consistency, it is best to use the same time period (three or five years) for a given type of vehicle for the entire analysis, unless there are major variations in terrain, etc. that would rationalize the use of different figures. If some of the data described above are not available, a rough estimate of annual vehicle capital costs can be obtained from local rates for hiring vehicles. In such a case, the cost of vehicles appears to be a recurrent, rather than a capital, item, but it should still be considered a capital cost.

Financial costs and economic costs should then be calculated as described in previous chapter (e.g. straight-line depreciation and economic calculation of capital) and form C3 should be completed, as described above for equipment.

The capital and recurrent costs of any vehicles purchased for the strategy should be added in the costing exercise. If the strategy opportunistically uses other vehicles that are available (e.g. borrowed from elsewhere), the actual expenditure incurred by using them for strategy activities should be added to the financial costs. Any economic analysis should include an adequate share of the capital and recurrent economic value of the use of these vehicles.

Allocation: If a vehicle is shared between implementation of the AIDS strategy and other work, the capital costs of that vehicle should be divided accordingly. See portion on allocation of running costs of vehicles in this chapter for suggested methodologies that can also be applied to the apportionment of their capital costs. The preferred method would be apportionment by mileage, followed by duration of vehicle use. It is necessary not to double count vehicles that travel between different organisational levels. For instance, if the cost of a vehicle is included at district level then none of its cost should be included at the field level to which it makes supervisory visits.

Suggestions regarding travel costs: Travel (other than by vehicles owned by the organisation) can also be classified as a separate category of costs. Some travel may not be done using vehicles belonging to the organisation, but rather by public transport (e.g.

taxis and by air). For instance, in community-based CSW peer education projects, field staff may often attend all educational sessions and travel by taxi to the sites. Travel should not be mixed up with vehicle cost, but rather included as an item under other recurrent costs (see section h). The total expenditure on travel should be added as part of financial costs. Economic costing is required if the price of this travel seems to be wrongly calculated.

If travel is included, it is important not to double-count its constituents under other categories (e.g. consultant's travel could be included here or under 'consultancy'; it is required that their travel be included under 'consultancy activities').

Strategy-specific Comments

(i) For HIV blood screening, vehicles used to conduct the strategy are likely to differ. Recruitment of donors at low risk of being HIV-infected may need mobile blood collection services. Reorganisation of services may necessitate additional transport for the central testing and subsequent distribution of blood.

(ii) For mass media and HIV education in schools, vehicles may be required during training activities and for the distribution of educational materials. Transportation costs may be comparatively high if printed IEC materials have to be distributed. This is not contracted out and hence costed as an aggregate input elsewhere.

(iii) In CSM, most transport needs, for instance for promotion or distribution activities, will usually be contracted out to other agencies. If the social marketing organisation owns and runs its own vehicles, an adequate share of the capital and recurrent costs of these should be apportioned to the CSM project.

(iv) For CSW peer education, vehicles may be needed by NGO staff to identify new project sites, hold education meetings and make supervisory and monitoring visits.

(v) Purchase of vehicles specifically for STD treatment is most common in vertical systems.

(vi) For VCT, vehicles may be used to take samples for testing, and to provide follow-up support to those tested.

(vii) For IDU interventions, means of transportation or travel may be utilized in training staff and volunteers, distribution of IEC and other supplies and safe disposal of contaminated supplies and equipment.

(d) Consultancies (Form C4)

Short-term consultancies can be considered as a separate input. Since many HIV prevention projects have been earlier set up vertically, they have been externally supported and are characterised by consultancy inputs provided by either expatriate or local experts. It is necessary to record these costs separately as they can be relatively high, generally financed in foreign currencies and may skew analyses if recorded as integral parts of other input categories. Consultancies may comprise of technical assistance from a variety of organisations, both national and international, for example from donor or specialized agencies or from advertising firms. Inputs may be given by consultants external to the implementing organisation or by experts from the organisation's own headquarters. The costs of consultancy packages usually includes salaries or fees, international and/or local travel and subsistence and sundry reimbursements. Some consultancies, such as those contributing to pilot projects or market research, will be given once only during project start-up and, if relevant to the analysis being undertaken, these costs should be recorded as capital costs on form C4. Start-up costs will be taken when analysis is of total costs of a project since inception but not included when analysis emphasizes on efficiency and sustainability of on-going activities. Some consultancies may not just be focused on the start-up phase but may instead be a capital component of the on-going project. Examples are training consultancies whose effects are anticipated to remain over several years. It is necessary to decide which consultancies to use, since different missions will have very different purposes. Where a project partly donor-financed there may be regular donor consultancies, especially for monitoring and evaluation purposes. The project itself may not incur financial costs for these inputs but, if they are considered essential for its local implementation, their economic costs should be added in any economic analysis.

It is recommended that cost be added where the consultancy forms a crucial part of project support, but excluded where it is for the purpose only of satisfying donor needs, for instance those monitoring or evaluation missions for the donor headquarters overseas. Long-term consultants, present for 12 months or more, should be recorded and costed on personnel form C5a. Consultancy inputs tend to differ considerably in terms of the number of individuals involved, the lengths of inputs and their purpose Column 1 of Form C4 can be used to list these details briefly, but adequately enough so as to distinguish the particular consultancy for future reference. The funder of the consultancy can be listed in column 2.

Financial cost: Generally only part of the costs of the consultancy package will be paid out from the project's in-country budget. Expatriate inputs, in particular, may be met by multi-or bilateral donors, at times even from non-project expenditure subheads. Only actual expenditure by the project requires to be recorded as a financial cost in Form C4. If a total expenditure figure is available for the consultancy, this can be listed directly in column 6 without being broken down into its component parts in columns 3, 4 and 5. The same method must be used for annual costing of capital consultancies as for other capital items. The number of years for which the effects of the consultancy are expected to remain should be listed in column 8. The total cost of the consultancy should be divided by the duration of effect, and the average annual cost should be listed in column 9.

Economic cost: The full value of the consultancy inputs (even if 'donated' from external funding) should be listed on Form C4 if the analysis is to use economic costs. Donors can be contacted for information on consultants' daily fees and subsistence rates and prices paid for air fares. Accurate information on these costs, often paid by headquarters offices overseas may not be available, but rough estimates should at least be found and listed in columns 3, 4 and 5. The total economic cost of the input should be listed in column 7. Where costs are met in foreign currency, this should be entered in a footnote and the local currency equivalent entered (see earlier sections on 'Currency' and 'Converting to constant prices'). Annualization of the costs of the consultancy must be done, with respect to other economic capital costs. The average annual economic cost should be listed in column 10.

Allocation: If the consultancy input is being divided between HIV prevention and other work, the costs of the input should be apportioned according to the consultants' time spent on each type of work. The allocated percentage and the resulting costs should be listed in columns 11 and/or 12.

Strategy-specific comments: Start-up consultancies, often used for training of trainers and the production of IEC materials, are necessary for many strategies. Although some governments or National AIDS Control Programmes may start IEC campaigns alone, mass media and CSW peer education projects are increasingly incurring consultancy costs particularly specially in the design and development of IEC materials. For HIV education in schools, some consultancy costs may be incurred in the design and development of the strategy and its syllabus and materials. CSM project are likely to have high start-up costs incurred by market research, project design and project launch. For STD treatment, some consultancies might give technical assistance for development of diagnosis and treatment protocols. Start-up consultancies may also initiate baseline studies to monitor different HIV prevention strategies, and be used for training of trainers and the production of IEC materials.

Recurrent Costs

Recurrent costs are costs for those inputs that are likely to be consumed (or replaced) within one year.

(e) Personnel (Form C5a)

"Salaries, wages, and other expenses associated with personnel are frequently the single largest cost item in health programmes. You should therefore take great care in estimating their value. In most cases, you will be interested in both the staff directly involved in the activity you are concerned with (e.g. nurses, health aides, trainers, supervisors) and other support staff (e.g. managers, administrators, cleaners, guards, drivers).

"The full cost of employing someone is represented by the individual's gross earnings-that is, the take-home pay plus any additional benefits, such as contributions to health insurance, social security, and pension plans, plus tax. These gross earnings should include any incentive payments, overtime, hardship bonuses, holiday and sick pay, and allowances for uniform, housing and travel. If the worker receives any additional commodities, housing or other non-monetary benefits, the value of these should also be estimated, using the prevailing prices of similar items (e.g. the current market rent for similar housing).

"*Sources of cost data:* Expenditure records and payrolls in the Ministry of Health will have cost data on salaries and allowances. You may need to look elsewhere for some data. For example, pensions may be paid by the Civil Service Board or another agency, and per diem allowances are often paid by external agencies. Data from the private market can help in the valuation of non-monetary benefits, such as housing. If you need to identify the earnings of particular individuals, ask for their salary grade rather than their actual salary. People are usually more reluctant to reveal their earnings than to state their position on a standard salary scale. Furthermore, it may be difficult to decide what the figure you are given means (gross or net salary, for example). Salary schedules can usually be obtained from the agency administering the civil service. Each type of information will need to be collected from the most appropriate level. If you ask only about salary grades, you will not get information about other allowances and bonuses. A rough estimate could be made by assuming that the average ratio between salaries and allowances for the whole institution (or a relevant subgroup) can-'be applied to each individual. For example, you may find from district-level expenditure data that allowances are, on average, about 12 per cent of salaries. You would then add an extra 12 per cent to-each individuals salary" (PHC: 35-36).

Financial cost: List, in column 1 of Form C5a, all staff who contribute to the activities of the strategy being costed, and notify in column 2, by whom they are being funded. Column 1 must comprise both voluntary and paid staff, and staff who are in support roles, as well as those directly implementing the strategy. In small-scale operations, this list can be by staff name and grade; in larger-scale operations, by staff category and grade. Information on gross earnings should listed in column 3. The mid-point of the salary range can be used where actual data are not available. An approximate financial value for all allowances and fringe benefits, whether received in cash or kind, should be entered in column 5. These may comprise, for instance, money payments for overtime or travel time, imputed rent for free accommodation, estimated cash values for uniforms or health care provided to staff. Salaries and allowances for long-term expatriate inputs should be differentiated from local salaries. Where these salaries and allowances are given in foreign currency, this should be noted in columns 5 and 6, and converted as described in the sections on 'Currency' and 'Converting' to constant prices' earlier on.

Short-term expatriate inputs should be noted as consultancies on Form C4 (capital) or C9 (recurrent). NGO service providers may make significant use of volunteers. Financial costs should include any incentives paid to them or benefits in kind. The costs of staff in other organisations to which strategy work is hired out may be added in fees charged to the lead organisation and should not be double-counted. Note that the forms are designed to gather annual personnel costs. If costs for an alternative time period are listed, this should be clearly indicated.

Economic cost: Since the long-term sustainability of depending on volunteers may not be ensured, a value for the time of volunteers should be added in the economic cost analysis. Volunteers could be questioned about their earning in the next most likely use of their time. In the case of volunteer workers or staff receiving token payments, a sample of such staff should be questioned about their earning in salaries and allowances in their next most likely use of time. This might vary from very little in areas of high unemployment, up to full salaries. This shadow wage should then be listed as an economic cost in column 4. In cases where expatriate inputs are being subsidized by part or full payment of salaries and allowances by external funders, the value of these subsidies should be added in the costs in columns 4 and 6. While estimating economic costs of expatriate inputs, thought should be given to whether an equally qualified national could be employed for the same work at a different cost. If this were possible, underneath the line stating the expatriate salary cost, state the cost of hiring a similarly qualified national. A sensitivity analysis could be carried out to assess the effect this change would have on the overall costs and cost-effectiveness of the project.

If it is thought that the salaries being given by the project are highly divergent from market trends, enquiries should be made locally about the market value of the work. For instance, civil servants may be overpaid through minimum wage agreements or underpaid compared with the private sector. In these cases, consideration should be given to substituting shadow prices for these inputs and listing them in column 4 (see the beginning of this chapter). In practice, the need to do this will rarely be faced and it should be carried out with care, as approximation of economic value of work can be difficult. For instance, an apparently underpaid government worker may work less hard or for fewer hours than his/her counterpart in the private sector, and so the salary given may, in fact, reasonably value the output of work.

Allocation: Some personnel may work fully for the HIV prevention strategy whilst others may divide their time between the strategy and other work. Personnel costs should be apportioned to the AIDS strategy according to time allocations. The suggested means of allocative time is to talk staff through the activities of their last working week, having ascertained that there was nothing out of ordinary about that week. If the earlier week had been special, for example a training week, the most recent special week should be chosen. Rather than using this prospectively, staff could be asked, to approximate retrospectively how they allocated their time. This might be most suitable for inputs of administrators and managers at the more central levels. At clinic and laboratory levels, personnel costs might be divided more accurately by activity measures (discussed as follows). If not included elsewhere, personnel costs of training activities should also be added. Costs should then be allocated according to time spent on HIV prevention as a proportion of total working time.

Time spent on general management and administration, breaks, sick leave, etc., should be allocated between the HIV prevention strategy and other work in the same ratio as specified working time. Worksheets to record the week under examination should be designed according to the nature of the working week in each situation (Such a worksheet is gives at Form C5b). The costs of personnel indirectly supporting the strategy, for instance receptionists and cleaners, should be allocated to the strategy on the basis of the average of the percentage allocations of other directly involved staff. If it is not possible to get time allocations for staff the next best alternative is to allocate their costs by activity allocations. For instance, the costs of National Blood Service laboratory technicians might be apportioned to the strategy according to the HIV tests as a percentage of total tests conducted. The ratio of personnel costs allocated to the AIDS strategy and the resulting costs should be listed in columns 9 and/or 10.

Strategy-specific Activities

(i) The following effects of the STD treatment for personnel costs should be analysed: the allocation of the costs of existing laboratory staff to HIV testing; the costs of any new laboratory staff hired to meet increased testing demand; allocation of the costs of existing health service staff for HIV activities such as pre- and post-test counselling; the costs of any additional staff for these activities; the cost of staffing any HIV-specific IEC material production/transmission and the personnel costs of collecting increased volumes of blood required due to increased levels of rejecting unsafe blood.

(ii) Mass media campaigns may invite inputs from celebrities to increase the popular appeal of their messages. Often these inputs will be given without charge and so are a zero financial cost for the strategy. An economic analysis should keep in wind whether free celebrity time is a practical assumption in the future of the project or in its replication elsewhere (whatever is the objective of the costing). If it is not viable, a shadow economic wage could be attributed to that input.

(iii) For HIV education in schools, it is necessary that the costs of all staff involved in the strategy be added. This comprises the cost of their time spent in training (initial training outside school, and follow-up training in the school), as well as the time that school staff members take in implementing the strategy.

(iv) Since the CSW peer education is labour-intensive, personnel costs are relatively high, or even the largest, proportion of total costs. There are two groups of personnel to be financed: community-level CSW peer educators and NGO staff based at the next level up. NGO staff like managers, field coordinators and supervisors will generally be full-time employees with formal salaries and allowances, the costs of which may require to be allocated between the strategy and other activities. The CSW peer educators may also get salaries and allowances or may 'work as volunteers, receiving only honoraria and reimbursement of expenses. In any economic analysis, a sample of volunteer workers should be questioned about their earning in the next most likely use of that voluntary time. A suitable shadow economic wage should then be calculated on the basis of their approximations and entered into the analysis. Peer educators may face losses of income (e.g. lower price of transactions due to use of condoms or due to marginalization because of their role as a peer educator). If approximate, this should also be evaluated and included in the shadow costings.

Suggestions on opportunity cost calculations of sex worker time

In Cameroon, it was hard to obtain a shadow wage for the volunteer time of peer educators, as they belonged to very varied backgrounds. However, when asked, "what did you give up?" The educators replied in terms of the loss of clients and lowering the price of the transaction, as they insisted on the use of a condom.

So as to get an estimate of the opportunity cost, the average loss of clients in a month was multiplied by the average price of a transaction. This average price was got by looking at the various sub-groups in the CSW population and the range of prices charged for a transaction.

Supplies (Form C6)

Supplies consists of materials that are used up in the span of a year. Equipment costing under $100 (unless national accounting procedures specify a different cutoff point) can also be considered as supplies even if they last longer than a year. All categories of supplies consumed should be noted in column 1 of Form C6 and their funding source listed in column 2. "You might wish to differentiate between supplies purchased from local currency and supplies requiring foreign exchange. The general data-handling process will be similar. In some cases, it will be important to identify separately, and summarize, major supply categories or categories of particular interest (i.e. calculate subtotals for drugs, stationery).

"The full cost of supplies should include the cost of transport to the point of use (i.e. any freight charges for import of materials and any internal distribution costs). The cost should be that of all the material consumed, including any that is lost or wasted as well as that which is actually used for its intended purpose. Losses can result from misplaced shipments, damage (e.g. from water or rodents), pilfering and materials becoming out of date. This loss has to be paid for by the programme, and should be included in the estimates. Supplies to be costed do not include those that are distributed but kept in store (as inventory stocks). Only those that are consumed should be counted.

"Unless expenditure records are very detailed, they are unlikely to be useful for estimating the costs of most of the materials specific to your programme. Instead, you will need information on quantities and prices.

"Quantities: For many supplies, there will be stores at different levels (national, regional, health centres), which will usually have their own inventory records. The quantity distributed from these stores during the year will be equal to the inventory at the beginning of the year plus the quantity received during the year less the inventory at the end of the year.

"The amount distributed is not necessarily the amount consumed: commodities may be stored at a lower level. Only at the lowest level of the distribution system, such as the health centre, are supplies dispensed the same as supplies consumed. However if you measure only consumption, you will fail to take into account the wastage that has occurred.

"Prices: Supply invoices, order forms, price lists and catalogues are sources of information about purchase prices or replacement prices. Costs of international and internal transport should be included. International freight costs can usually be readily determined (supply invoices and order forms should include them) and should not be overlooked, since they often add a further 10-20 per cent to the original price. it may be more difficult to estimate internal transport costs; in fact, if supplies are transported by vehicles belonging to the programme, the costs will be included in the vehicle running costs and should not be included here" (PHC: 36-38).

Financial Cost: If detailed expenditure records are there, the financial costs of supplies consumed should be listed directly in column 6. These costs should comprise transportation of the supplies to the point of use. Where accurate expenditure records are not available, costs should be calculated from quantities consumed, including loss and wastage (column 3), and unit costs (column 4/5). If quantities consumed are not given, it may be required to estimate consumption based on output. For instance, to approximate the consumables used in blood collection and testing an inventory of all the consumables needed per unit of blood could be made, and then multiplied by the number of units collected. Allow a margin (approx. 10 per cent) for loss and wastage.

Imported supplies should be classified together and, where purchased in foreign exchange, this should be listed in a footnote on the form. The equivalent local currency costs should be calculated using the procedure outlined in 'Currency' and 'Converting to constant prices' earlier on in this chapter. Remember that if materials have a life of more than a year (e.g. a film), then their value will need to be annualized over their length of life, and these materials should be treated as capital items.

Economic cost: Market prices should be considered as the economic unit costs of donated goods and these prices should be entered in column 5. Where market prices for certain supplies are known to be highly divergent from the actual opportunity costs, a shadow price should be substituted as the economic cost in column 5 or 7. This may be specially relevant in the case of drug and condom supplies where import prices may be subsidized, inflated due to economic/political tying to certain exporters, or manipulated through unrealistic exchange rates. Shadow prices can be found from the international market prices or can be calculated from the Essential Drugs Programme or from a supplier such as UN Supplies Division and converted into local currency prices using the market exchange rate.

Allocation: Data, especially when taken from expenditure records, may aggregate supplies consumed by HIV prevention and other work. It may, therefore, be important to apportion only a part of the costs of the supplies to HIV prevention. This would generally be done on the basis of activity measures as shown in some of the examples in Part 3. The percentage allocation of costs and the resultant cost to the strategy should be entered in column 8 and/or 9:

(i) Additional supply costs will be incurred for HIV blood screening. These will comprise one-test kits, small pieces of equipment, and chemical reagents for use in the laboratories. There may also be an increase in the cost of medical and surgical equipment for collecting blood, such as blood bags and needles, since a greater volume of blood will require to be collected to allow for rejecting. Some office supply costs might also increase, in line with increased strategy-related administration.

(ii) For mass media and HIV education in schools; if the lead organisation is producing some of its own IEC materials then significant supply costs may be incurred directly for such commodities like photocopying supplies, ink, videos, cassettes and batteries or, indirectly, through the use of government printing facilities. Alternatively, IEC material production may be contracted out and costed as an aggregate activity. For instance, commercial printers may be used to make campaign posters and pamphlets and specialized advertising agencies may be used to produce television and radio materials.

(iii) The recurrent costs of CSM projects can be heavy and this is, in part, due to the costs of the condom supplies. Their source and price can be highly diverse. The financial cost of the condoms should be found and, if imported, this should comprise the cost of transportation into the country. The financial price of condoms may be highly inflated or subsidized. Inflated prices occur when donor's commodities are bought from home markets and are considerably more costly than those on the international market. The financial cost to the project may be zero if the commodities are donated but the financial cost to the donor may be more than the economic opportunity cost of those commodities.

(iv) Many CSM projects get condoms from donors and their supply prices are more than prices on the international market. If there is a possibility that, in the future, condoms bought at competitive prices will be provided to the project, then a shadow economic price could be used in the cost analysis. An adequate price can be obtained from the Essential Drugs Programme or from a supplier such as UN Supplies Division. In truth, however, many social marketing projects will continue to be sourced with donors' condoms for the foreseeable future and the increased prices may, therefore, be most suited for any medium-term analysis of these projects.

(v) Where the project is able to negotiate with commercial condom suppliers to provide subsidized condoms in return for financing some of their marketing and promotion activities, there may again be a need to calculate a shadow economic price for the costing analysis. This is specially true if the present subsidized price cannot be guaranteed in the future.

(vi) Supplies for STD treatment will mainly comprise diagnostics, laboratory supplies, condoms and drugs. Costs of these are likely to be comparatively high and should therefore, be calculated with some care. Costs of some supplies may require to be allocated between STD and non-STD work and this should be done according to the activity measures discussed in the personnel section earlier in the chapter.

(vii) To list the quantity and cost of drugs consumed by an STD clinic, expenditure information should be seeked from the next organisational level up-say, the district level-where cost and quantities may have already been combined and recorded in accounting information. If that information is not available, drug use should be examined at the clinic in question, for instance from their inventories. In both these situations, drug costs may need to be apportioned between treatment of STD and other illnesses. If neither of the above methods is possible, clinicians could be asked to note their prescriptions prospectively over a period of, say, one week. Total STD drug costs could then be approximated from average prescription costs and facility utilization data. The total costs got this way should be inflated by a locally agreed factor to allow for the additional costs of drug wastage and loss.

Suggestions on calculating the total costs of drug in an STD treatment programme in the United Republic of Tanzania

The quantity of drugs prescribed was approximated through the analysis of a sample of health units. Data on drugs prescribed for the last 20 registered STD cases were listed from a survey of treatment registers. The drugs prescribed were costed from unit prices provided by the national Essential Drugs Programme in the United Republic of Tanzania (inclusive of cost, insurance and freight). Then the total cost of drugs supplied was approximated on the basis of the total number of STD cases seen in all the health units and an estimate of the proportion of patients actually supplied with drugs. Since drugs are often in short supply, it was estimated that only 40 per cent of patients were supplied drugs (with sensitivity analysis of 20 per cent and 60 per cent used). Costs of drug storage and delivery within the country were estimated roughly as a cost per health unit (multiplied by the number of health units) and then added to the total drug costs.

(viii) The main supply costs for CSW peer education, will be for IEC materials and for condoms. The relatively high recurrent costs of the strategy can, in part, be assigned to condom supplies, the source and price of which can be highly diverse.

(g) Vehicle operation and maintenance (Form C7)

Many health programmes depend on vehicles to distribute supplies, allow coordination and supervision, and otherwise conduct the provision of care. Often, transport is a weak link;

vehicles are there but fail to operate efficiently because of deficiency of fuel or spare parts. It is important to know what it costs to operate and maintain vehicles. Unfortunately, these costs are among the most difficult to ascertain. The costs of operating, maintaining and repairing vehicles must be measured. These will comprise materials, such as fuel, lubricants, insurance and registration fees, tyres, batteries and spare parts. The cost of drivers should be listed under 'personnel'.

If a mechanic is hired for the programme, the cost will also be added under 'personnel'. However, where repairs and maintenance are contracted out, or where they are done by a different office or agency, their cost should be added under 'vehicle operating costs' (i.e. you should make an approximation of total repair costs, including an allowance for the mechanic's salary, rather than including the salary under personnel costs).

"Expenditure records may give some indication of the cost of operating and maintaining vehicles, but it is likely that you will need to interview drivers and mechanics and consult logbooks to get a sufficiently detailed picture. Fuel consumption is one input for which records are probably reasonably good. If not, you should be able to estimate fuel consumption based on the mileage of the vehicle. Logbooks should indicate distance travelled (say, 5000 kilometres), and drivers should be able to tell you the average distance travelled per litre of fuel consumed for that particular type of car in the prevailing conditions (say, 10 km per litre). Total consumption is then 5000/10 = 500 litres. The price paid per litre for fuel multiplied by the number of litres used gives the total cost of the fuel (even if it is merely charged to a government account). If logbooks and other information sources are not adequate for the calculations suggested (which is all too often the case), alternative data sources can probably be employed. For example, your ministry's central motor pool personnel may be able to give you a rough estimate of the total annual cost of operating and maintaining each type of vehicle. With information on the vehicles used (and the fraction of their time devoted to your programme) you can make a 'rough and ready' calculation that will suffice.

"Oil and filter changes and other maintenance may be done irregularly or on a routine basis, either after a set number of kilometres or at regular time intervals (e.g. once a year). If you are unable to calculate these inputs in the same way as fuel, you could simply increase fuel costs by a set percentage (e.g. 15 per cent) to allow for them. Again, the central motor pool may help you with this" (PHC: 39).

Financial cost: Form C7 summarizes the main resources for operating, maintaining and repairing project vehicles. The simplest and preferred method is to access expenditure records for vehicle running costs. If such expenditure records are not there, logbooks and staff interviews should be used. If logbooks are not available, staff interviews alone will have to give the necessary information. If no accurate information can be collected from any of the above, the least preferred method is to use the value of standard government mileage allowances to the mileage undertaken in implementation of the strategy. These mileage allowances are supposed to reimburse officers for official use of private vehicles or to charge them for private use of official vehicles and are understood to cover running costs plus depreciation. In this situation it is necessary to ensure that the capital costs of the vehicles are not double-counted between this form and Form C3.

Economic cost: Where financial costs are visibly different from opportunity costs, for instance, where mechanics work voluntarily on vehicles, approximate economic costs can be listed in column 4. Where vehicle running costs are a relatively small component of overall costs, limited time should be taken trying to calculate economic costs and shadow prices.

Allocation: Some vehicles may be used exclusively for conducting the AIDS strategy. Others, however, may be shared between the strategy and other work and their running costs must be divided accordingly. In columns 5 and 6 of Form C7, the allocation made can be noted and used to apportion cost. It is suggested that all inputs on Form C7, apart from personnel, be allocated by mileage undertaken for the strategy as a proportion of total mileage in a sample month. If logbooks are not there from which to get this information, staff should be questioned to ascertain the proportion of days in a sample month that the vehicle is used to implement the strategy. The way in which all the above allocations are made should be listed either as a footnote on the worksheet or separately.

(h) Building operation and maintenance (Form C8)

"Operation and maintenance of inputs is quite easily handled.' Although observers are sometimes concerned with utility expenses, these do not form a large proportion of the total. If it is difficult to obtain information, draw on past experience (and other opinions) to obtain a rough estimate of building operation and maintenance as a proportion of the annual market rent. Multiply the annual rent by this proportion to obtain an amount for operation and maintenance.

"Operation and maintenance for buildings should include charges for lighting, water, telephones, heating, insurance, cleaning materials, painting, and repairs to plumbing, roofing, heating and office furniture. As previously noted, the salaries of guards, cleaners, etc. should be counted under 'personnel'.

"This is one category where recorded expenditure data are sometimes quite adequate. Recurrent costs for buildings will normally be listed under such headings as 'utilities, maintenance or cleaning, and security'" (PHC: 40).

Financial cost: If expenditure information is attained, then it should be used to fill Form C8. Information should ideally be listed for a full year to permit for seasonal fluctuations in utility expenditure. If annual utility expenditure figures are available, then a total figure can be noted for the year in row 15 rather than being built up by month. If expenditure information is not there, then a percentage of the rental value of the building should be used to cover these costs. The appropriate percentage should be approximated by local managers and will differ according to the quality of building construction, the age of the building and the nature of the services being provided there. The figure calculated should be listed in row 16 of Form C8, alone with an explanatory footnote. This rough approximation is acceptable, as these costs are unlikely to be significant in the overall profile of costs.

Economic cost: If it is thought necessary substitute any shadow prices for financial costs, clear footnotes should indicate where and why this has been undertaken.

Allocation: If a building is shared between HIV prevention and other work, the running costs of that building will have to be allocated accordingly. This should be done by calculating the ratio of floor space used by the HIV-related work as a proportion of the total floor space of the building that the running costs are incurred in, and/or by the proportion of time that that space is used for the HIV work. The percentage allocation of costs and the resulting cost to the strategy should be entered in row 17.

(i) Short-term consultancies (recurrent) (Form C9)

An explanation of short-term consultancy inputs, in section (d) under 'Capital costs' above has been made. Under recurrent costs consultancy inputs that recur all through the life of the project should be listed, for instance, consultancy inputs to annual monitoring and review missions. It should, however, be made assessed as to whether such consultancies are a crucial and necessary part of the progress of the project, in which case they should be included, or whether they are implemented for donors' own monitoring purposes and should be excluded from the costs of the project.

Financial cost: See section (d) above. How often the consultancy inputs are being costed should be listed in column 8 of Form C9. (If a project document is available, this should give the planned frequency of these inputs.) The frequency of the inputs may point out the need to translate costs noted for one particular year into average annual costs. For instance, if consultants are provided for monitoring missions every other year, the costs for each mission should be halved to provide an average annual cost. Average annual costs can then be listed in columns 9 and/or 10.

Economic cost and Allocation: See section (d) above.

(j) Other recurrent costs (Form C10)

"This is the residual category. It was recommended that all the inputs to training and social mobilization programmes should be added together to give a single figure, rather than including them under separate headings (personnel, buildings, etc.). Each of these input categories has its recurrent counterpart, when activities are repeated periodically. The sum of these activities over one year is a recurrent cost of the programme. There are probably no special problems involved, or instructions needed, for calculating the costs of these two categories of inputs. If a training or social mobilization programme serves more than one programme, the total cost should be distributed among those served. If training and social mobilization are costed as discrete inputs, care must be taken not to duplicate any of the costs elsewhere in the exercise.

"Recurrent equipment costs include fuel (e.g. kerosene for cold-chain refrigerators) or electricity operating costs (but only if these are not included under building operation and maintenance), as well as the cost of spares for maintenance and repairs. Other categories might include postage, printing, photocopying and the costs of operating and maintaining equipment, but not stationery, which is counted under 'supplies'.

"Expenditure records may contain some data, but they are unlikely to be detailed enough. For a piece of electrically operated equipment you will need to know its power requirements (the number of kilowatt-hours), the length of time it is operated over the year, and the cost per unit of electricity. You will probably need to ask the people directly responsible for the equipment about the kind of maintenance and repairs that were necessary and what spare parts were needed. There are a variety of 'rules of thumb' to estimate the likely operating and maintenance costs of equipment used in health programmes. Most of these rules relate recurrent costs to the original capital expenditure. The specific relationships will depend on the price structure in the country, the nature of the equipment, and so forth. You should explore the precise cost relationships in your own situation rather than relying on approximations from elsewhere" (PHC: 40-41).

For most HIV prevention strategies, this cost category will be comparatively insignificant. It will, however, be more significant for mass media and condom social marketing strategies as media costs will be included here. How these are treated is discussed further under the following 'strategy-specific comments'. Potential inputs for other strategies include equipment maintenance, operating and repair costs, postage, photocopying and printing. Only minoı attempts should be made to cost these inputs where they are likely to be negligible in the overall composition of costs.

Financial cost: If available, cost information should be taken from expenditure records. If unavailable, rough approximation of costs should be made from quantities of inputs used and prices.

Economic cost: If any of the financial prices visibly do not reflect opportunity costs, a shadow price should be substituted in column 4, but attempt in doing this should be proportional to the cost. Media fees are treated separately on the following paras.

Allocation: Shared costs should be allocated in a manner appropriate to the way that they are incurred. The percentage allocation of costs and the resulting cost to the strategy should be listed in column 5 and/or 6.

Strategy-specific Comments :

(i) In HIV blood screening, where blood donors are given money as incentive, there may be higher payments, for larger volume of blood collected. Same applies also to any refreshments or gifts provided for blood donors, and should be counted as other recurrent items.

(ii) For mass media and CSM, this category of costs will comprise the costs of media time and/or space. Seeing from the trends of other public health media campaigns, it can be expected that media costs will differ greatly between countries. This indicates absolute and relative differences in the price of media, which affects the project's purchasing power, and also variations in the type and quality of media used.

(iii) In countries having state-run newspapers and radio and television channels, the financial costs of using them may be subsidized or made free to the project. In some countries, it may even be mandatory that a certain percentage of air time or press space is to be dedicated to educational messages. If it is thought that this situation cannot be ensured in the future, then any economic analysis should add the economic opportunity cost of the media used. This is best found by ascertaining the cost of the same amount and quality of media time or space for a commercial campaign.

(iv) Where media slots are rated at a commercial price to the project, it can be taken that these costs are economic ones, including all associated costs and overheads.

(v) For HIV education in schools and CSW peer education,

where expenditure for initial or refresher training is found, it is possible that training costs will be a substantial part of total costs. The training packages may comprise the costs of preparation, the venue used, transport, materials, trainers' personnel costs, per diems of attendees and the cost of the time of the school staff participating.

(k) Private costs (Form C11)

Private individuals have been taken as a source of funds in this chapter. Each of the 'C' Forms solicits information on the source of funds for inputs, and the fact that some inputs are privately financed can be listed there. Eventhough these guidelines take the perspective of service providers, these expenditures should be listed in order to calculate project revenues and hence the net costs of the project.

Form C11 gives a separate record of the cash fees that are charged from individual clients. The form is very general, allowing collection by month for a number of types of fees and will, therefore, need to be suited to particular circumstances. The preferred method of obtaining the data is from fee collection registers or income records. If these are not available, approximation of fees raised should be made from number of clients and average official fee rates, although these approximations will clearly miss over- and under- charging and any leakage of funds. Data on fees paid should be kept separate and not included in total costs (otherwise there will be double-counting). To set the data in context, more qualitative information should also be listed on how the fees are charged and managed; for example, whether they can be kept at the level at which they are collected and what they can rightfully be used for.

- For HIV blood screening, the most common private costs will comprise fees paid for transfusions. Data on fees collected should be collected from the BTS. However, it may be possible only to record gross fees for the transfusion provided, and not to disaggregate the element of the overall fee that patients are understood to pay for 'HIV-safe' blood.
- Private individuals may fund some of the supply inputs,

for instance by providing their own needles and blood bags. These costs can be included to the costs that the BTS itself incurs, since they buy additional resources required to implement the strategy.

- Individuals may meet some costs to receive mass media messages and information. These costs may comprise batteries to operate radios, television licence fees and the price of newspapers and magazines. However, receiving the HIV/AIDS messages will be only a small percentage of the benefits of subscribing to these forms of media. It is suggested that, even when a societal viewpoint is being taken, these user costs be excluded. Private travel costs linked with the strategy should be least since, almost by definition, mass media bring the messages and information to the population wherever they are. Time may be spent hearing HIV prevention material on the radio or television, or reading IEC material in the press. It is suggested, however, that the economic opportunity cost of that time be assumed as being zero.
- HIV education in schools makes use of an available audience. It can be assumed that school students do not incur any additional financial, time or travel costs to participate in the HIV/AIDS education sessions.
- For CSM, the main type of private expenditure will be for the buying of condoms. Total private expenditure will be a factor of the marketing prices at retail outlets and the amount of sales. Where the price of condoms is standard throughout the country, it will be simpler to derive this figure than in situations where retailers are free to set their own profit margins. Private time and travel costs will also be spent in obtaining the condoms and this could be examined if costing from a societal perspective. From a provider perspective, the relevant information will be the net sales revenue given back to the centre rather than private costs at the periphery. The social marketing organisation should be able to give information on net sales revenue. This is subtracted from project costs to obtain total net costs.

- For STD treatment, the most frequent private costs will be fees paid for consultation and/or drugs. Similarly, in VCT, fees may be paid for testing. Information on fees gathered should be available from the service provider, sometimes collected at a more central level than the clinics themselves. The degree to which total fees collected can be equated with fees paid will partly depend on the amount of leakage of funds from the system. Fees given to service providers should be identified separately if all inputs provided at the facility have already been costed. They can be minused from total strategy costs to give net costs.
- If drugs are prescribed but not given by the clinic itself, the cost of buying the drug will also fall upon clients. If the costing study is from the providers perspective, then these costs can be overlooked. If private costs are to be included, the costs of these drugs should be examined. Clients could be interviewed for information on their expenditure or, in another option, prospectively collected clinicians' prescriptions for STD treatment could be used to approximate the average costs of obtaining these prescriptions from pharmacies.
- CSW peer education projects may charge CSWs for some of the services offered; for instance, fees may be charged for condoms. In such a situation, the implementing NGO should be able to give information on the quantity of sales and unit prices. The establishments within which the project is conducted may also be charged fees — for instance, a flat fee for being incorporated in the project, or fees for educational talks given to their CSWs. Again, the NGO should have records of these private costs. These fees can be minused from total project costs, to arrive at net total costs.

Collection of Outcome Data

During the process of collecting data on costs, data on the outputs and results of the programme should also be gathered, so as calculate average and unit costs of the strategy. Unless you participate in model-based evaluations or clinical trials, it is only adequate to try and obtain process and intermediate measures of outcome.

These outcomes will vary according to the HIV prevention strategies used (e.g., for CSM projects you may be seeing the number of condoms sold, on the other hand in VCT projects you could use the number of people counselled and tested as the outcome measure). Even if you are trying to find a number of methods which are being used together, the use of process or intermediate outcomes means that the measures will be relatively special to each strategy.

So as to decide for which outcome measures you will try and gather data, it will be necessary to ask the following questions:

(a) What is the main purpose of the project or strategy?
(b) What are the main activities in the project or strategy?
(c) What are the outputs of the project or strategy? Are they connected to particular activities?
(d) What are the main intermediate outcomes?

The answers to the questions will help find out the nature, of the outcome measures for the entire project as well as by activity. They will facilitate in classifying the type of data that needs to be collected both for process and intermediate outcomes. In practice, data availability will substantially influence the actual measures that can be used in the cost analysis. However, before beginning the data collection, it is necessary to understand the nature of both process and intermediate measures.

Process Measures of Outcomes

These measures are used to record the outputs of the project or programme. To determine the outputs it is useful to review the individual activities. For example, in an IDU needle exchange project, the activities include development of IEC materials, recruitment of volunteers, training of staff, exchange of needles, disposal of needles and counselling. Given these activities, we can think of a number of output measures:

- number of materials produced (e.g. printed matter, books)
- number of volunteers trained
- number of staff trained
- number of condoms distributed
- number of needles/syringes exchanged or distributed
- number of people reached

A measure of output that can provide more information about the possible impact of the project is:

- number of persons in contact with NEP and exchanging needles

It is generally easy to obtain process measures of outputs from programmes. The data are often routinely measured and available from existing project or programme records. Thus the important thing is to identify the range of activities and consider the individual outputs that are associated with them.

Intermediate Measures of Outcome

These measures reflect intermediate changes needed to achieve health impacts of the prevention strategy. However, several of these variables are continuous (e.g. frequency and sharing, proportion of sex acts in which condoms are used). This raises a number of issues about the extent to which you indicate a change has occurred (e.g. do you include someone who has reduced injection frequency or increased condom use frequency by 1 per cent?). Is there a threshold or critical value above which we consider that people have modified their risky behaviour? If we converted these measures to percentage variables such as:

- percentage of IDUs sharing syringes
- percentage cleaning syringes with disinfectant
- frequency of use of a single syringe,

a unit cost calculation would then make no sense (e.g. cost per percentage of IDUs sharing syringes).

A comprehensive intermediate outcome measure would be the number of people who have reduced risky behaviour. This could be a summation of all those who both stop sharing syringes and reduce their frequency of IDU.

Thus, for instance, in a mass media campaign, a process outcome consists of the number of radio messages produced by the intervention. For the campaign to change health status (e.g. contain HIV infections), people require to be exposed to the campaign and messages so as to change behaviour. In this case, an intermediate outcome could be the number of people accessed by the radio message. For HIV education in schools, an intermediate outcome would consist of the number of students who are taught the curriculum. Data for intermediate outcomes are more difficult to find than simple output information. These outcomes may not be systematically monitored, and you may have to depend on project evaluations to help produce approximation of likely ranges of values for your intermediate outcome measures.

Multiple and non-discrete outcomes

There are multiple interventions and multiple outcomes connected with many prevention interventions. Apart from lowering the risk of HIV transmission, some interventions can also decrease the risk of other STD, pregnancies, blood-borne infections such as hepatitis B and C, and reduce death due to overdoses. In presenting the costs of the different HIV prevention strategies, the direct and indirect benefits of the strategy should also be listed.

Cost Analysis

Now that the component costs have been collected, the data requires to be aggregated or collated. Sheets C1-C10 permit you to collect costs at different levels. Form B is a summary of costs at each level. Once this is over, all the levels can be added up and listed in Form A — the Project Summary sheet — to arrive at total costs.

Adding up Costs

Those projects using a computer can enter data directly into a spreadsheet package using the Microsoft Excel spreadsheets found on the UNAIDS website (www.unaids.org/publications) or the CD-ROM: *Economics in HIV/AIDS planning: getting priorities right* UNAIDS (June 2000). They would be recommended to apply the same approaches to enable collation of data from Forms C onto summary forms A and B (World Health Organisation also provides such software(9). If a computer is not available, data can be collated manually. Form B (collating all Form C data at a particular organisational level) can be completed with either financial or economic costs, or both. The Base Year costs in the final column or row of each Form C should be listed in their appropriate rows on Form B and then all of the input categories added up to give a total cost of the AIDS strategy at that organisational level. It must be kept in mind that if only a sample of units had been costed to stand for all units at a particular level, it is the total cost of the population of units from which the sample was found that should be calculated and transferred to Form B. A record should be made of this calculation.

Form A collates the costs from each organisational level (the Form B data) to arrive at the overall cost of the HIV prevention strategy or programme. Form A can be completed with either financial or economic costs (completing a form for each, if needed). If the set of B forms shows all costs at all organisational levels, then they can be summed together to arrive at the overall total cost. If, however, the strategy being costed is only part of a larger programme, then it may be required to allocate only a proportion of higher-level costs to the overall cost calculation. For instance, we may be concerned about costing an AIDS strategy in one district only, within a region of 10 districts and a country of 20 regions. In this case, if costs were apportioned equally between sub-units at a particular organisational level, Form A would need to collate 100 per cent of the costs calculated for the district, 10 per cent of the costs calculated for the region and 5 per cent of the costs calculated for the central level. Only these required proportions of costs at each organisational level should be transferred to Form A for the final summation. If it is visible that sub-units (for instance, districts or regions) do not make equal demands on the level above, it may be decided to make a more accurate allocation of costs, for example weighted by share of total budget or number of staff per sub-unit. A clear record should be made of how this proportion was derived, both in footnotes on the forms if they are being compiled manually and also more formally.

Cost Profile

Once Form A is filled, to you have more or less made a cost profile of the project or programme that you have examined. It will look like the table as follows:

Cost Category	*Annual Cost (currency)*	*Total Cost (%)*
Capital		
Buildings	5000	10
Equipment	5000	10
Vehicles	5000	10
Consultancies (non-recurrent)	0	
Total Capital Costs	**15000**	**30**
Recurrent		
Personnel	20000	40
Supplies	5000	10
Vehicle operation and maintenance	5000	10
Building operation and maintenance	1000	2
Consultancies (recurrent)	4000	8
Other	0	
Total Recurrent Costs	**35000**	**70**
Total Costs	**50000**	**100%**

Source: PHC: 12.

You could also obtain a cost profile in terms of activities rather than inputs. These profiles are useful in pointing out major cost components (and thus identifying possible areas where improvements in efficiency may have significant impact on costs). For instance, high drug cost could mean wastage. These cost profiles can be compared across varied projects and programmes, as well as within programmes. Within programmes the profiles can be presented by different delivery units or providers, and a comparison can be made between them. "If there are significant differences in cost profiles, then this may mean that there may be ways to re-structure and improve efficiency" (PHC: 13). However, comparison of cost profiles across countries or regions is difficult because of different price structures. Comparison of cost profiles over time could be more useful than the comparison across different projects. Thus, one must be careful while generalizing from cost profiles, and that too when appropriate.

Unit costs

Once total costs figures of a programme or project have been arrived at, then unit costs can be derived. These can be calculated in terms of the outcome indicators for which you have gathered data in sheet D, and are simply calculated as total costs divided by the outcome measure. Unit costs can be used to compare costs between similar projects, and determine issues of project efficiency. There are many factors affecting unit costs, they include the following:

(i) different prices paid for inputs by projects in different locations;

(ii) different input mixes used by different projects (e.g. more staff or more supplies);

(iii) different levels of staff efficiency;

(iv) efficiencies could be gained due to the size or scale of the project (economic of scale). For instance, condom social marketing projects seem to have lower unit costs in countries with large populations;

(v) efficiencies could be gained due to having a number of services or projects undertaken together (economies of scope).

Nevertheless, not all differences in unit costs should be attributed to variations in efficiency. A higher unit cost may not indicate a less efficient programme. There may be other factors driving these differences, for instance:

(a) Differences in unit costs may mean differences in ease of delivery of services. For instance, a project that is based in rural areas with a more dispersed population, or projects reaching more marginalized groups, might entail higher costs. Thus there may be equity factors for allocation of more resources to this project.

(b) The time taken by a project or programme may affect unit costs. While comparing an established programme with a relatively new programme consideration should be given to this. This is specially true for CSM projects, where some projects have gone from start-up to accruing profits in the span of 12-15 years.

Along with this, you may want to obtain unit costs by activity. For instance, if you have the costs of IEC production within a condom social marketing programme and the number of IEC materials produced, then you can find out the unit costs of the materials produced. If training is an activity, then you can produce the unit cost per training session. This can enable analysis of efficiency of particular activities within a project

Making Use of Cost Analysis in Planning and Budgeting

Once the basic cost analysis is complete, the information can be used in many ways to aid planning and budgeting for the future. In general, current cost data can serve as a baseline for arriving at information for both the future and for other projects. What is clearly required is to consider to what extent the project from which you are obtaining cost information is similar to the activities that you wish to do. The financial cost analysis can help in understanding of budgeting requirements of a specified project. The financial cost analysis will give you an idea of the total resources that have been spent. The financial analyses will also serve as a baseline for future budgeting. There are many ways that you can use existing cost data to help in budgeting:

(a) An ingredients approach would imply that you note down all of the possible inputs and then determine to what degree you will be using them in the future project for the expected level of output (e.g. number of persons counselled) that you would like to achieve. Once you have considered the 'quantity', you can then work out the price and the cost. For instance, if you think that you will need 1.25 nurses, you can determine whether to hire one full-time nurse and one part-time nurse, or whether it is more practical to hire one nurse and pay for extra hours put in. This approach needs a lot of detailed cost information and is appropriate if programme conditions are changing quickly.

(b) A less detailed approach to budgeting would entail taking the current costs of a project, according to your own circumstances, and then do a rough adjustment depending on how similar you think the projects are. An important factor to determine is whether the project you are taking the costs from is actually running successfully, Alternatively, you could apply some mark-up to the costs (e.g. 20 per cent) to allow some margin of error.

Irrespective of the method you use, if you are budgeting for the future you require to adjust the price or cost information for inflation, You will require to determine what level of inflation to take into account, and that prices will rise every year. So, for example, in a country with a relatively stable level of inflation of 8 per cent, you may choose 10 per cent as the proportion by which you expect prices to increase each year. However, if you are in an environment with rapid inflation, you may desire to convert your costs to a more stable currency such as the US dollar and then do your budget calculations.

Financial cost analyses will also facilitate in considering the affordability of projects, as they provide information on the amount of money that is needed to run a project. This information can be used to determine the range of sources and funds that are available to finance the project.

However, financial cost analyses only reflect the actual expenditure on a project. If a project had substantial donated components, then depending on financial cost analyses will give a wrong view of the actual resources being used. Thus when determining issues such as replication of projects to different settings or scaling-up projects in size, it is crucial to determine what basic infrastructure may have been in place which was not accounted for in a financial cost analysis. For instance, many NGO-based projects often get assistance in the start-up phase (e.g. exchange of goods. in kind or subsidized printing). It is here that economic analyses are useful

Annex 1

Data Collection Sheets

This annex contains the data collection sheets, which are arranged as follows:

1. Background data sheet

2. Form A — Project Summary sheet—presents costs by input and level. This is a collation of all Form B summary sheets.

3. Form B - Summary of costs at each level. This is a collation of all Forms C1 - C10.

4. Forms C1 - C10 provide the basis for data collection by input category:
   CI — capital costs: buildings
   C2 — capital costs: equipment
   C3 — capital costs: vehicles
   C4 — capital costs: consultancies
   C5a — recurrent costs: personnel
   C5b — example of personnel time allocation form
   C6 — recurrent costs: supplies
   C7 — recurrent costs: vehicles operation and maintenance
   C8 — recurrent costs: building operation and maintenance
   C9 — recurrent costs: consultancies
   C10 — recurrent costs: other
   C11 — cost recovery: private costs

5. Form D — collection of output/outcome data

Background Data Sheet

Country ....
Project ....
Local currency ....
Discount rate (for base year) .... Source ....

Consumer Price Indices (CPI) for years spanned by data collection:

Year	....	CPI	....
	....		....
	....		....
	....		....

Market Exchange Rates for years spanned by data collection:

		$	Other
Year	....	....	....
	....	....	....
	....	....	....
	....	....	....

Official Exchange Rates for years spanned by data collection:

		$	Other
Year	....	....	....
	....	....	....
	....	....	....
	....	....	....

Local Market Interest Rates for years spanned by data collection:

Year	....	....
	....	....
	....	....
	....	....

Local Official Interest Rates for years spanned by data collection:

Year	....	....
	....	....
	....	....
	....	....

FORM A
PROJECT SUMMARY SHEET
(Collation of all Form 'B' summary sheets)

Country ....

Project ....

Local currency ....

Costs for Base Year ....

Financial costs / economic costs (delete as applicable)

Cost Category	*Level*	*Level*	*Level*	*Total cost (%)*
Capital				
Buildings				
Equipment				
Vehicles				
Consultancies (non-recurrent)				
Total Capital Costs				
Recurrent				
Personnel				
Supplies				
Vehicle operation and maintenance				
Building operation and maintenance				
Consultancies (recurrent)				
Other				
Total Recurrent Costs				
Total Costs				

FORM B
SUMMARY OF COSTS AT EACH LEVEL
(Collation of Forms C1 - C10).

Country ....

Project ....

Project Level ....

Local currency ....

Costs for Base Year ....

Cost Category	*Financial costs*	*Economic costs*
Capital		
Buildings		
Equipment		
Vehicles		
Consultancies (non-recurrent)		
Total capital costs		
Recurrent		
Personnel		
Supplies		
Vehicle operation and maintenance		
Building operation and maintenance		
Consultancies (recurrent)		
Other		
Total recurrent costs		
Total costs		

Once all the component costs have been collected, then the data need to be aggregated or collated. Sheets C1 - C10 allowed you to collect costs at different levels. Form B is thus a summary of costs at each level. Once this is done, all the levels can be added up on Form A-the Project Summary sheet.

FORM C1
CAPITAL COSTS: BUILDINGS

Country .... Cost Data Collected from months ....

Project .... Source of Data ....

Project Level .... Chosen Base year ....

Buildings (list)	*Funded by*	*Annual rent/hire*		*Furni-shing @ 10%*	*Total cost*		*(% allocation)*			
		Fin.	*Ec.*		*Fin. (3+5)*	*Ec. (4+5)*	*Fin.*	*Ec.*	*Fin.*	*Ec.*
(1)	(2)	(3)	(4)	(5)	(6)	(7)	(8)	(9)	(10)	(11)
Total										

FORM C2
CAPITAL COSTS: EQUIPMENT

Country .... Cost Data Collected from months ....
Project .... Source of Data ....
Project Level .... Chosen Base year ....
Local currency ....

Equipment (list)	*Funded by*	*Cost*		*Life expectancy or working iife*	*Annual cost*		*(% allocation) Cost*		*Base Year Cost*	
		Fin.	*Ec.*		*Fin.*	*Ec.*	*Fin.*	*Ec.*	*Fin.*	*Ec.*
(1)	(2)	(3)	(4)	(5)	(6)	(7)	(8)	(9)	(10)	(11)
Total										

FORM C3
CAPITAL COSTS: VEHICLES

Country .... Cost Data Collected from months ....

Project .... Source of Data ....

Project Level .... Chosen Base year ....

Local currency ....

Vehicles (list)	*Funded by*	*Cost*		*Life expectancy or working life*	*Annual Cost*		*(% allocation) Cost*		*Base Year Cost*	
		Fin.	*Ec.*		*Fin.*	*Ec.*	*Fin.*	*Ec.*	*Fin.*	*Ec.*
(1)	(2)	(3)	(4)	(5)	(6)	(7)	(8)	(9)	(10)	(11)
Total										

FORM C4
CAPITAL COSTS: CONSUL TANCIES

Country .... Cost Data Collected from months ....

Project .... Source of Data ....

Project Level .... Chosen Base year ....

Local currency ....

Consultancy detail	*Funded by*	*Fees*	*Travel*	*Subsistence + misc*	*Total Cost (3) + (4) + (5)*		*Life of effect*	*Annual cost*		*(% allocation) cost*		*Base Year cost*	
					Fin.	*Ec.*		*Fin.*	*Ec.*	*Fin.*	*Ec.*	*Fin.*	*Ec.*
(1)	*(2)*	*(3)*	*(4)*	*(5)*	*(6)*	*(7)*	*(8)*	*(9)*	*(10)*	*(11)*	*(12)*	*(13)*	*(14)*
Total													

FORM C5a
RECURRENT COSTS: PERSONNEL

Country .... Cost Data Collected from months ....
Project .... Source of Data ....
Project Level .... Chosen Base year ....
Local currency ....

Category of personnel (list with grade where appropriate)	*Funded by*	*Gross annual salary*		*Cost of annual allowances (specify)*		*Total annual cost*		*(% allocation Cost*		*Bae Year Cost*	
		Fin.	*Ec.*	*Fin.*	*Ec.*	*Fin.* (3)+(5)	*Ec.* (4)+(6)	*Fin.*	*Ec.*	*Fin.*	*Ec.*
(1)	(2)	(3)	(4)	(5)	(6)	(7)	(8)	(9)	(10)	(11)	(12)
Total											

FORM C5b
EXAMPLE OF PERSONNEL TIME ALLOCATION FORM

Country .... Cost Data Collected from months ....

Project .... Source of Data ....

Project Level .... Chosen Base year ....

Local currency ....

Time/Day									12		1		2		3		4		*Total strategy hours*	
Mon																				
Tues																				
Wed																				
Thur																				
Fri																				
Sat																				
Sun																				
Total Hours																				
Percentage of hours																				

List time allocation by arrows as indicated:

——HIV prevention strategy work; - - - - Non-HIV prevention strategy work.

FORM C6
RECURRENT COST: SUPPLIES

Country .... Cost data collected from months ....

Project .... Source of data ....

Project Level .... Chosen Base year ....

Local currency ....

Supplies (list)	*Funded by*	*Quantity consumed (including loss and wastage)*	*Unit Cost*		*Cost*		*(% allocation) Cost*		*Base Year Cost*	
			Fin.	*Ec.*	*Fin.* (3)×(4)	*Ec.*	*Fin.*	*Ec.*	*Fin.*	*Ec.*
(1)	(2)	(3)	(4)	(5)	(6)	(7)	(8)	(9)	(10)	(11)
Total										

FORM C7

RECURRENT COSTS: VEHICLE OPERATION AND MAINTENANCE

Country .... Cost data collected from months ....

Project .... Source of data ....

Project Level .... Chosen Base year ....

Local currency ....

Supplies (list)	*Funded by*	*Cost*		*(% allocation) Cost*		*Base Year Cost*	
		Fin.	*Ec.*	*Fin.*	*Ec.*	*Fin.*	*Ec.*
(1)	(2)	(3)	(4)	(5)	(6)	(7)	(8)
Petrol/diesel							
Oil							
Maintenance							
Insurance							
Registration							
Repairs							
Spare parts							
Total							

FORM C8
RECURRENT COSTS: BUILDING OPERATION AND MAINTENANCE

Country .... Cost data collected from months ....
Project .... Source of data ....
Project Level .... Chosen Base year ....
Local currency ....

(1) Utility	*Telephone/fax*	*Insurance*	*Maint./repair*	*Other*
(2) Source of funds				
(3) January				
(4) February				
(5) March				
(6) April				
(7) May				
(8) June				
(9) July				
(10) August				
(11) September				
(12) October				
(13) November				
(14) December				
(15) Annual cost				
(16) Total annual cost				
(17) (% allocation) cost				
(18) Base Year cost				

FORM C9
RECURRENT COSTS: CONSULTANCIES

Country .... Cost Data Collected from months ....

Project .... Source of Data ....

Project Level .... Chosen Base year ....

Local currency ....

Consultancy detail	*Funded by*	*Fees*	*Travel*	*Subsistence + misc*	*Total Cost (3) + (4) + (5)*		*Frequency*	*Annual Cost*		*(% allocation) Cost*		*Base Year Cost*	
					Fin.	*Ec.*		*Fin.*	*Ec.*	*Fin.*	*Ec.*	*Fin.*	*Ec.*
(1)	(2)	(3)	(4)	(5)	(6)	(7)	(8)	(9)	(10)	(11)	(12)	(13)	(14)
Total													

FORM C10
RECURRENT COSTS: OTHER

Country .... Cost data collected from months ....

Project .... Source of data ....

Project Level .... Chosen Base Year ....

Local Currency ....

Input (detail)	*Funded by*	*Annual Cost*		*(% allocation) Cost*		*Base Year Cost*	
		Fin.	*Ec.*	*Fin.*	*Ec.*	*Fin.*	*Ec.*
(1)	*(2)*	*(3)*	*(4)*	*(5)*	*(6)*	*(7)*	*(8)*
Total							

FORM C11
COST RECOVERY: PRIVATE COSTS

Country	....	Cost data collected from months	....
Project	....	Source of data	....
Project Level	....	Chosen Base Year	....
Local Currency	....		

Fee type (specify)				
January				
February				
March				
April				
May				
June				
July				
August				
September				
October				
November				
December				
Annual Total				
Strategy Total				
Base year Equivalent Value				

FORM D
OUTPUT/OUTCOME DATA

Country ....

Project ....

Outputs for Base year ....

Indicators	*Units*	*Quantity*
Process Indicators		
Intermediate Indicators		

Eleven

Greater Involvement of People Living with or Affected by HIV/AIDS (GIPA)

The HIV/AIDS pandemic has been rapidly increasing all over the world. Knowing fully well its deadly consequences and threat to the whole world there was an urgent need to mobilize international support to fight against this epidemic. It was felt important to make fight against AIDS a part of national agenda. To this effect the 1994 Paris AIDS Summit was held where, 42 national governments assembled and declared that the principle of greater involvement of people living with or affected by HIV/AIDS (GIPA) is crucial to ethical and effective national responses to the epidemic (See Annexure). This is, thus, the official position of these government, which have committed themselves to supporting full involvement of persons living with or affected by HIV/AIDS (PWHAs)[1] in the "common response to the pandemic at all-national, regional and global-levels". Precious little has been so far to make this principle a reality. Rather than being taken up by those for national responses, GIPA has been most strongly advocated by individuals living with or affected by HIV/AIDS, often by "going public" about their serostatus in order to give a human face and voice to the epidemic. At times, several major constraints do arise.

Constraints of GIPA

(a) GIPA is not represented in national policies and programmes in any concerted or large-scale way, and there is an almost total absence of mechanisms allowing or encouraging PWHAs' experiences, perception and skill to be considered (much less utilized). This is mainly because no major global, regional or national campaigns have yet been initiated to raise awareness and understanding of GIPA.

(b) Social, cultural and political situations, often marked by high levels and denial, fear and stigmatization, are contrary to the involvement of PWHAs.[2]

(c) PWHAs are often in stressful position, economically weak and having no structure that allows them to contribute to policy changes.

(d) Both PWHAs and existing AIDS Programme managers and staff need education and skill-building SO as to enable GIPA have its optimum impact. No single method of implementing GIPA can be successful give these different challenges, as well as particular local ones in different places. In spite of this sufficient experience has been gathered around the world to give guidance on how GIPA can be effectively translated into action.

What Does GIPA Do?

GIPA (Greater Involvement of People Living with or Affected by HIV/AIDS) at its best performs two important functions:

(a) recognizing the important contribution people challenges by HIV/AIDS can make in the response to the epidemic.

(b) creating an environment within society for their involvement and active participation in all aspects of that response.

This contribution can be made at all spheres, from the individual to the organisational, and in all sectors from the social and cultural to the economic and political, The Paris declaration specifically emphasizes the role of networks of PWHAs and community-based organisation.

Who are the people living with or affected by HIV/AIDS (PWHAs)?

The original term used in the declaration, "people living with HIV/AIDS", has since been enlarged by broad consensus to the term "people living with or affected by HIV/AIDS" (PWHA). It is important to recognize that PWHA is not a single class of persons but a continuum. The continuum runs from individuals living with the symptoms of AIDS, on the one hand, to HIV-negative partners, family members and close friends of HIV positive persons on the other.

The Meaning of "Greater Involvement"

There is noting better than direct experience, which can be considered a kind of expertise if accompanied by the skill to communicate well. As its best, therefore, greater involvement by PWHAs means creating a space for individuals to:

(a) use their observations of living with or being affected by HIV/AIDS in the greater response to the epidemic.

(b) give a human face and voice to the epidemic in the minds of people not directly affected by it.

Operationally this involvement may (and should)! Include varied roles at many different levels, For instance, participation of PWHAs is already acknowledged to some degree at the international level multilateral institutions and in regional and international conferences, at the national level in national AIDS programmes, and at local level in the community-based associations which often implement prevention, care and support activities very often the roles open to PWHAs at all of these levels are limited to observer or educational functions. Figure 1 shows a model of ways in which people living with or affected by HIV/AIDS can play a much wider range of roles. It should be clear that the model does not include an important part of GIPA which includes efforts of individuals at a personal level.

Although not part of any formal agreement or structure, a major portion of the worldwide response to HIV/AIDS is the work of individual people caring - in many different ways - for their seropostive family members and friends. It is also the work of people who, by "living positively" or openly interacting with PWHAs, act as examples to others, thereby contradicting both the denial and stigma that attend the epidemic in many communities. It should be highlighted, however, that GIPA does not necessarily mean disclosing one's serostatus. Although there should be nothing to stop PWHAs declaring their serostatus openly to their colleagues and community, PWHAs also have the right to decide to be involved without making their serostatus public. In other words, GIPA cannot be reduced to "no visibility = no involvement".

This pyramid models the increasing level of involvement advocated by GIPA, with the highest level representing complete application of the GIPA principle. Ideally, GIPA is applied at all levels of organisation.

Decision Makers: PWHAs participate in decision-making or policy-making bodies, and their inputs are valued equally with all the other members of theses bodies.

Experts: PWHAs are recognized as important sources of information, knowledge and skills who participate - on the same level as professionals - in design, adaptation and evaluation of interventions.

Implementers: PWHAs carry out real but instrumental roles in interventions, e.g. as careers, peer educators or outreach workers. However, PWHAs do not design the intervention or have little say in how it is run.

Speakers: PWHAs are used as spokesperson in campaigns to change behaviours, or are brought into conferences or meetings to "share their views" but otherwise do not participate. (This is often perceived as "token" participation, where the organizers are conscious of the need to be seen as involving PWHAs, but do not give them any real power or responsibility.)

Contributors: activities involve PWHAs only marginally, generally when the PWHAs is already well-known. For example, using an HIV-positive pop star on a poster, or having relatives of someone who has recently died of AIDS speak about that person at public occasions.

Target Audiences: activities are aimed at or conducted for PWHAs, or address them en masse rather than as individuals. However, PWHAs should be recognized as more than (a) anonymous images on leaflets, posters, or in information, education and communication (IEC) campaigns, (b) people who only receive services, or (c) as "patients" at this level. They can provide important feedback which in turn can influence or inform the sources of the information.

Fig. 1: A Pyramid of involvement by PWHAs

Why Involve PWHAs?

There are many reasons why GIPA is so necessary as a response. To the epidemic. At the social level, public recognition of involvement helps reduce stigma and discrimination, and sends a message to society regarding acceptance and recognition of the importance of PWHAs. Within organisations, involvement can be an important tool for breaking down barriers, whether subjective or objective. Organisations comprise individuals, and individuals who are neither infected nor affected by HIV/AIDS often have preconceived notions which are seriously misinformed about PWHAs. Not surprisingly, these notions can be reflected in organisational policies or practices, even when the organisations are actively involved in the response such as government ministries, international agencies or NGOs. Discrimination against PWHAs is widespread, though it is largely ingenious or hidden, and is not even always consciously acknowledged as such by those who discriminate.

Working with seropositive individuals on a daily basis, and having a name and face to relate with the concept of "a person with HIV and AIDS" - where previously the association was with a virus or terrible disease - helps people fight against their fears and prejudices, and change their perception of PWHAs. By giving a basis for partnership, mutual respect and understanding, GIPA breaks down simplistic concepts of " service giver" (that is, the person who is not HIV-positive) and " service receiver" (the person who is HIV positive). Other than reducing discrimination , GIPA can strengthen an organisation or activity by exposing it to the unique perspectives that PWHAs' direct observations can bring. This reinforcement can be at the level of general morale and team-building, or it may include substantial improvement in the way an organisation actually works. For example, PWHAs can perform. An indispensable support function in an organisation or activity that has employed designated "AIDS workers" such as public health educators, clinicians, psychologists and social workers. Even though workers often get little emotional or practical support for their AIDS prevention and education activities, PWHA's can supply the benefit of their knowledge, help instill confidence in them reassure them to the importance of their contribution. Finally, GIPA is advantageous for PWHAs as individuals. Experience demonstrate that this kind of involvement - especially if it comes after a period of hopelessness and depression - build up a person's motivation. PWHAs (like everyone else) need to feel valued for what they can offer. Involvement give HIV-positive people support and empowers them in ways that increases the value of their contribution to the organisation or activity.

Obstacles to Implementing GIPA at Higher Levels

Other than promising a range of potential benefits, GIPA undergoes a number of challenges, particularly at higher levels of organisations. These include:

(a) Difficulty of declaring HIV Status Publicly

Declaring one's own serostatus to family, community or workplace is more difficult in some countries or cultures than others. In some cases, precautions are necessary to protect who disclose their positive serostatus, since this can create serious consequences for them in their jobs and within their families and communities. Discrimination comes about in different ways, from almost invisible types of social behaviour on the one hand, to physical violence on the other. Similarly, PWHAs fears may range from purely personal (and not always accurate) feeling of discrimination all the way to objectively based fears of rejection and violence.

(b) Lack of Organisations Collaborating with PWHAs

There are presently too few organisations involving or collaborating with PWHAs in their day-to-day work. This may be because of absence of awareness or information among those in charge of the organisations, or it may be due to active discrimination or unconscious prejudice. Lack of awareness or information is a particular difficulty within the private sector: Management is often wholly unaware of the possible affect of the epidemic on their economic performance, and does not understand the possible benefits of GIPA.

(c) Absence of skills and preparation for PWHAs

Absence of skills can create a variety of obstacles. Firstly, not all are born with the natural potential to speak about issues like sexuality and health - it is a skill that most often has to be learned. Secondly, facing a possibly aggressive or uncomprehending environment can lead to the "burnout" affect unless a person is either very strong to start with or has undergone an empowerment process. Due to these reasons, communication and personal empowerment counselling should form part a generic training package for people participating in GIPA initiatives. Such training must also be reinforced by ongoing support for PWHAs if their effectiveness is to remain high and their motivation strong. Thirdly, special orientation or job-specific training may be needed to make up for the lack of particular technical skills or knowledge. The point raises the question of appropriate hiring. Clearly, hiring people specifically because they are HIV-positive, and without regard to their particular skills and capabilities, is symbolic, it puts the emphasis on the virus rather than on the person and his or her character and abilities. At the same time, those responsible for employing should acknowledge the value of the PWHA's experience-based expertise and include this in their decision-making.

(d) Absence of proper environment for HIV-positive people within organisations

Organisations may not have a proper policy for the employment or involvement of people living with HIV and AIDS. They may also not have the sort of environment and facilities that are important or helpful to seropositive people like: health care facilities, medical insurance and psychosocial support.

(e) Question of Sustainability

It has to be acknowledged that HIV- positive people may fall sick due to their infection and its related illnesses, and that some of them may even die. This poses a challenge particularly to the private sector, in which employers may feel threatened by reduced working hours due to illness and loss of skilled manpower due to untimely death. Obviously, the possibility of falling sick or dying exists for all employees or members of organisations, whatever their serostatus; the odds are greater for people living with HIV/AIDS than for many other groups of people. This issue should not be ignored, since it is real. Instead, it has to be discussed in order to pre-empt difficulties with sustainability.

Countering the Challenges

Observations have shown that there are a number of effective ways to deal with the above-mentioned challenges to implementing or modifying proving GIPA initiatives.

(a) Document existing observations and inculcate lessons learned

The results of many accomplished GIPA-related interventions have been published. These are very helpful in explaining the concept and its benefits, as well as providing solid examples of how interventions can be implemented. Prominent examples include the following :

The AIDS Services Organisation (TASO), Uganda. Much of the organizing urge which created and shaped TASO was provided by a woman whose husband had died of AIDS. Her major skill was not formal training but rather her strong commitment which resulted from her personal experience of caring for a person with AIDS and her exposure to HIV-related stigma. From its inception in 1988, TASO developed into one of the most important and innovative groups in the AIDS field internationally.[3]

Asia Pacific Network of People living with HIV/AIDS (APN+)

This promoting organisation had its beginnings in February 1994 when 42 PWHAs from 8 countries in the ASIA Pacific region met in Kuala Lumpur, Malaysia. They agreed to exert influence for the betterment of PWHAs in the region, and of work against stigma and discriminations. APN+ now includes 10 countries. (See the internet location http://www.hivnet.ch/gnp/asp1.html)/

The "UNV Support to People Living with HIV/AIDS" Project

This is a combined pilot project between the United Nations Development Programme (UNDP), United Nations Volunteer

Programme (UNV), UNAIDS and the Network of African People. Living with HIV and AIDS (NAP+). Presently in its second year of operation in Malawi and Zambia, and soon to be extended to Asia, the project recruits, trains and supports HIV-positive persons whom it places as National UN Volunteers in different host institutions.[4]

(b) Create a More Helpful and Supportive Environment

GIPA cannot have its full impact or be widely applied until there are changes in wider society, with discrimination and stigma transformed into tolerance and acceptance by information and awareness drives. Political, traditional and religious leaders have a large role to play by bringing about these social changes. Parliamentarians, for instance, can help draw up antidiscrimination laws and national policies on AIDS and the workplace. At a separate level, law enforcement officers in some societies can do much to prevent physical violence and other forms of threats against PWHAs. Such official activities by these prominent individuals, as well as less formal participation in local efforts dealing with AIDS in their communities can have a large impact on overall social attitudes to people living with or affected by HIV/AIDS. Social change must be matched by institutional change in international, national, or local organisations. A number of initiatives can be taken to help HIV seropositive individuals to take part in the response to the epidemic. However as mentioned under the challenges, it is the absolute right of people to choose not to divulge their serostatus or their relationship to somebody infected by HIV.

(c) Understand the Requirements and Worries of the Private Sector

In parts of the world hardest hit by the epidemic, many businesses have large numbers of employees infected or affected by HIV/AIDS. Due to this, the private sector has both a strong interest and a major role to play in the reaction to the epidemic. It is therefore extremely important for businesses and their leaders to accept that, while AIDS among employees and the general public can affect productivity and profitability, constructive measures can be taken that will minimise such adverse effects. GIPA is at the core of such measures.

An important message for business leaders is that PWHAs can be ideal partners to plan for comprehensive prevention, care and support interventions at the workplace. For example, peer education by someone infected with HIV or someone "with AIDS in the family" can be part of a corporate action plan. Other GIPA-related activities which can be carried out or supported by the private sector include: taking out advertisements stating that HIV-positive people are invited to apply for employment with the company; giving counselling services at her workplace; having senior management collaborate continuously and publicly with PWHAs in creating HIV/AIDS workplace plans; giving training and adapting workload for PLWHAs engaged in the workplace plan.

All such activities have their costs and must be budgeted for, but none is highly costly and their cost-benefit ratio is generally very favorable. Anything that is regarded as "preferential hiring" is potentially controversial. In the private sector - as much or more so, than in the public or nongovernmental sectors - hiring should be largely based on qualification for nay given job. However, this should not be used as a reason for refusing to hire a PWHAs who can (a) sufficiently fill a specific job's requirements and (b) provide the important benefits of GIPA. Experience shows that PWHAs very often have very strong commitment which can justify their being hired before they have all the technical expertise require by the job (although, clearly, this expertise is expected to be acquired eventually, either through training or on-the-job experience). Examples can be found in the work of many parents and partners of HIV-positive people: without any training administration or management, and with extremely limited resources, these "HIV-affected" people have been able to arrange and run thousands of support and advocacy groups around the world. Such strong commitment, which can also highlight or enhance the personal charisma of certain individuals, can be an important resource when channelled by GIPA into other organisations and activities.

(d) Training and Ongoing Support for Individuals

GIPA activities cannot rely indefinitely on individuals commitment or charisma; however, it is very important to provide training and support for PWHAs actively engaged in the response to the epidemic. International organisations and associations for persons living with HIV/AIDS can help to provide a generic package for those individuals wanting to divulge their personal relation to AIDS. As well as training for the specific job, GIPA training packages for PWHAs should include:

(i) personal empowerment;
(ii) communication and presentation skills;
(iii) HIV/AIDS knowledge;
(iv) legal aspects of HIV/AIDS;
(v) skills for organizing and conducting policy dialogue.

If the employee is given administrative responsibility for GIPA activities, training should also involve the basics of programme planning and monitoring.

(e) Training and Orientation for Organisations

It is equally necessary that organisations - including top executives as well as supervisory staff - get the benefit of training and orientation according to the rules of GIPA. Among other issues, host organisations must be aware that by hiring a person living with HIV they have an added responsibility with ethical consequences. This responsibility is not difficult to take on if carried out with proper preparation.

This training should be carried out at least in three parts:

(i) challenges and benefits of instituting GIPA and recruiting PWHAs, including policy formulation
(ii) responsibilities of, and implementation strategies for, host organisations
(iii) lessons learned from existing GIPA efforts (best practice).

All of this should be targeted at creating supportive environments as well as organisational structures which permit the full application of GIPA at the highest levels.

ANNEXURE I

Declaration of the Paris AIDS Summit

1 December, 1994

(Note: statements directly related to GIPA have been italicized)

We the Heads of Government or Representatives of the 42 States assembled in Paris on 1 December, 1994:

I. Mindful that the AIDS pandemic, by virtue of its magnitude, constitutes a threat to humanity, that its spread is affecting all societies that it is hindering the social and economic development, in particular of the worst affected countries, and increasing disparities within and between countries, that poverty and discrimination are contributing factors in the spread of the pandemic, that HIV/AIDS inflicts irreparable damage on families and communities, that the pandemic concerns all people without distinction but that women, children and youth are becoming infected at an increasing rate, that it not only causes physical and emotional suffering, but is often used as a justification for grave violations of human rights,

   Mindful also that obstacles of all kinds - cultural, legal, economic and political - are hampering information, prevention, care and support efforts, that HIV/AIDS prevention and care support strategies are inseparable, and hence must be an integral component of an effective and comprehensive approach to combating the pandemic, that new local, national and international forms of solidarity are emerging, involving in particular people living with HIV/AIDS and community based organisations,

II. Solemnly declare our obligation as political leaders to make the fight against HIV/AIDS a priority, our obligation to act with compassion for and in solidarity with those with HIV or at risk of becoming infected, both within our societies and internationally, our determination to ensure that all persons living with HIV/AIDS are able to realize the full and equal enjoyment of their fundamental rights and freedoms without distinction and under all circumstances, our determination to fight against poverty, stigmatization, and discrimination, our determination to mobilize all of society - the public and private sectors, community-based organisations and people living with HIV/AIDS - in a spirit of true partnership, our appreciation and support for the activities and work carried out by multilateral, intergovernmental, non-governmental and community-based organisations, and our recognition of their important role in combating the pandemic, our conviction that only more vigorous and better coordinated action worldwide, sustained over the long term - such as that to be undertaken by the joint and co-sponsored United Nations programme on HIV/AIDS - can halt the pandemic,

III. Undertake in our national policies to protect and promote the rights of individuals, in particular those living with or most vulnerable to HIV/AIDS, through the legal and social environment, fully involve nongovernmental and community-based organisations as well as people living with HIV/AIDS in the formulation and implementation of public policies, ensure equal protection under the law for persons living with HIV/AIDS with regard to access to health care, employment, travel, housing and social welfare, intensify the following range of essential approaches for the prevention of HIV/AIDS:

- promotion of and access to various culturally acceptable prevention strategies and products, including condoms and treatment of sexually transmitted diseases,
- promotion of appropriate prevention education, including sex and gender education, for youth in school and out of school,
- improvement of women's status, education and living conditions,
- specific risk-reduction activities for and in collaboration with the most vulnerable populations, such as groups at high risk of sexual transmission and migrant populations,
- the safety of blood and blood products,
- strengthen primary health care systems as a basis for

prevention and care, and integrate HIV/AIDS activities into these systems, so as to ensure equitable access to comprehensive care,

- make available necessary resources to better combat the pandemic, including adequate support for people infected with HIV/AIDS, nongovernmental organisations and community-based organisations working with vulnerable populations.

IV. Are resolved to step up the international cooperation through the following measures and initiatives. We shall do so by providing our commitment and support to the development of the joint and co-sponsored United Nations programme on HIV/AIDS, as the appropriate framework to reinforce partnerships between all involved and give guidance and worldwide leadership in the fight against HIV/AIDS. The scope of each initiative should be further defined and developed in the context of the joint and co-sponsored programme and other appropriate fora:

1. Support a greater involvement of people living with HIV/AIDS through an initiative to strengthen the capacity and coordination of networks of people living with HIV/AIDS and community-based organisations. By ensuring their full involvement in our common response to the pandemic at all - national, regional and global - levels, this initiative will, in particular, stimulate the creation of supportive political, legal and social environments.
2. Promote global collaboration for HIV/AIDS research by supporting national and international partnerships between the public and private sectors, in order to accelerate the development of prevention and treatment technologies, including vaccines and microbicides, and to provide for the measures needed to help ensure their accessibility in developing countries. This collaborative effort should include related social and behavioural research.
3. Strengthen international collaboration for blood safety with a view to coordinating technical information,

proposing standards for good manufacturing practice for all blood products, and fostering the establishment and implementation of cooperative partnerships to ensure blood safety in all countries.

4. Encourage a global care initiative so as to reinforce the national capability of countries, especially those in greatest need, to ensure access to comprehensive care and social support services, essential drugs and existing preventive methods.
5. Mobilize local, national and international organisations assisting as part of their regular activities children and youth, including orphans, at risk of infection or affected by HIV/AIDS, in order to encourage a global partnership to reduce the impact of the HIV/AIDS pandemic upon the world's children and youth.
6. Support initiatives to reduce the vulnerability of women to HIV/AIDS by encouraging national and international efforts aimed at the empowerment of women: by raising their status and eliminating adverse social, economic and cultural factors; by ensuring their participation in all the decision-making and implementation processes which concern them; and by establishing linkages and strengthening the networks that promote women's rights.
7. Strengthen national and international mechanisms that are concerned with HIV/AIDS related human rights and ethics, including the use of an advisory council and national and regional networks to provide leadership, advocacy and guidance in order to ensure that non-discrimination, human rights and ethical principles form an integral part of the response to the pandemic.

We urge all countries and the international community to provide the resources necessary for the measures and initiatives mentioned above.

We call upon all countries, the future joint and co-sponsored United Nations programme on HIV/AIDS and its six member organisations and programmes to take all steps possible to implement this Declaration in accordance with other multilateral and bilateral aid programmes and intergovernmental and non-governmental organisations.

Countries which were represented at the Paris Summit and signed the Declaration:

Argentina, Australia, Bahamas, Belgium, Brazil, Burundi, Cambodia, Cameroon, Canada, China, Cote d'lvoire, Denmark, Djibouti, Finland, France, Germany, India, Indonesia, Italy, Japan, Mexico, Morocco, Mozambique, Netherlands, Norway, Philippines, Portugal, Romania, Russian Federation, Senegal, Spain, Sweden, Switzerland, United Republic of Tanzania, Thailand, Tunisia, Uganda, United Kingdom, United States of America, Viet Nam, Zambia, Zimbabwe.

Notes and References

1. The Global Network of Persons Living with HIV/AIDS (GNP+) and the International Community of Women Living with HIV/AIDS (ICW) have officially adopted the acronym PWHA to designate people infected with or affected by HIV/AIDS. This includes people who are seropositive and the people who surround them (such as loved ones, parents and friends).
2. The Uganda musician Philly Lutaaya was the first African celebrity to disclose his HIV-positive status and to join the campaign against AIDS. An early advocate of "living positively" and eliminating stigma, he is considered one of the "fathers" of GIPA. Philly Lutaaya died in 1989.
3. For more information, see Hampton J. Living positively with AIDS available from Teaching Aids at Low Cost (TALC), London, United Kingdom.
4. See Enhancing the Greater Involvement of People Living with HIV and AIDS (GIPA) in sub-Saharan Africa: A UN Response: How far have we gone? UNDP, in press.

Twelve

Implementing PRSPs Under HIPC Initiative

Object of Study

Since HIV/AIDS has become a well acknowledged threat to development in many developing countries, these countries attempted to "mainstream" HIV/AIDS into instruments of development. For poor countries, the PRSPs serve as the country's agenda for poverty reduction, they have become an important instrument for country-level managers and analysts to make objective proposals for the inclusion of HIV/AIDS in the poverty reduction effort.

The study undertaken in this section will enable country officials and their partners to prepare and negotiate effectively the inclusion of enhanced HIV/AIDS programmes in their PRSPs (Poverty Reduction Strategy Papers) and instruments of debt relief under the intensified HIPC (Heavily Indebted Poor Country) initiative. The PRSPs document country-owned strategies for poverty alleviation and provide the basis for a wide range of development programmes to be financed from public funds and grants. A PRSP provides a basis for concessional lending by international financial institutions in case of countries intending to implement the programme. The enhanced Heavily Indebted Poor Country (HIPC) Initiative adopted by the Boards of the World Bank and IMF in 1999 was initiated with the object of accelerating the delivery of HIPC Initiative assistance thus linking debt relief more firmly and transparently to poverty reduction. Simultaneously, the enhancements more than doubled the amount of relief projected to be provided under the Initiative. It is expected through this that external debt servicing will be cut by approximately

US$50 billion. When combined with traditional debt relief, the initiative will reduce by more than two-thirds the outstanding debt of more than 30 countries.

While several countries have initiated HIV/AIDS alleviating efforts effectively, many have yet to do so. For countries that are eligible for debt relief through the enhanced HIPC initiative, there is a possibility for significant increases in the public financing of HIV/AIDS programmes through earmarking of funds. Only a few countries thus far have taken this opportunity. This study is intended to assist countries seeking to develop effective sections on HIV/AIDS in their PRSPs and HIPC documents.

Purview of Study

It is addressed primarily to those with responsibilities for - or interest in - getting the HIV/AIDS agenda into the broader development efforts of each country. While including analysts and policy-makers in National AIDS Commissions or similar cross-sectoral bodies, Ministries of Finance/Economic Development and nongovernmental organisations at the country level, it also has officials of agencies that work with countries on PRSPs and HIPC documents, including NGOs, the international financial institutions, United Nations agencies with a remit that includes poverty reduction and development, foundations and bilateral development agencies in its purview.

Links Between HIV/AIDS and Poverty

The study addresses two sets of issues:

(a) AIDS as a cause of poverty or AIDS deepening poverty and

(b) the combined effect of poverty and income inequalities on social transactions - including sex, patterns of vulnerability and patterns of risky behaviour in relation to HIV infection and AIDS.

Figure 1 shows the links between AIDS and poverty. A detail on this account is given in Annexure 1.

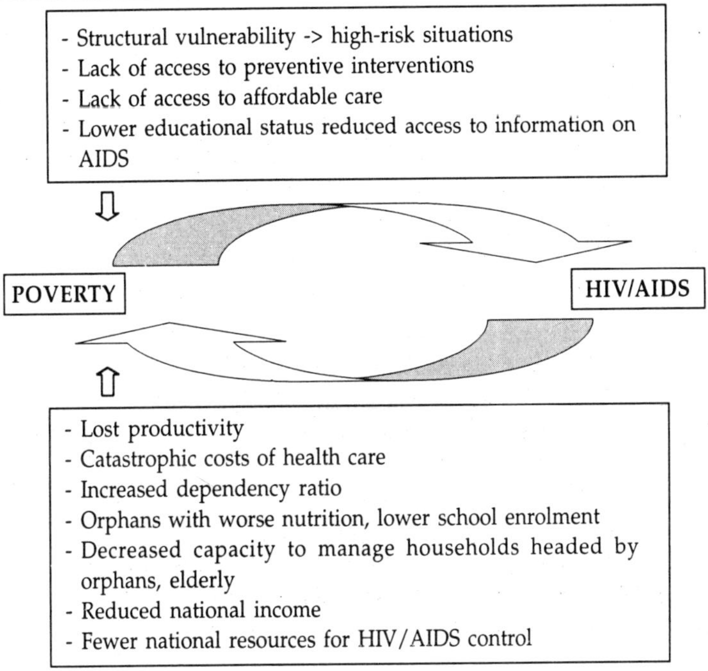

FIGURE 1: RELATIONSHIP BETWEEN POVERTY AND HIV/AIDS: A SIMPLIFIED VIEW

AIDS Effect on Poverty

(i) Reduction in income and increased medical expenses

Surveys show that households suffer a significant decrease in income and huge rises in medical care spending which further leads to fewer purchases, diminished savings and dissavings.

(ii) Reduction in agricultural output and increased medical expenses

In a study in Thailand, one-third of rural families affected by AIDS experience a halving of their agricultural output. Another 15 per cent had to withdraw their children from schools, and over half of the elderly people were left to take care of themselves. The last year of an AIDS patient's life entailed an expenditure of US$1000 on medical care the equivalent of an average annual income.

(iii) Halving of education and food consumption alongwith multiplication of health expenditure

The outlay on school education was halved; food consumption went down by almost half per capita and expenditure on health more than quadrupled. When family members in urban areas fall ill, they often return to their villages to be looked after by their families, thus adding to the pressure on already scarce resources and increasing the probability of a spouse or others in the rural community of being affected.

(iv) Growth in number of orphans and decrease in their schooling chances

The number of orphans grows and the number of potential caregivers declines. The traditional coping mechanisms are utilized to breaking point. Households headed by orphans are becoming common in high-prevalence countries. In Uganda, with the death of one or both parents, the chance of orphans going to school is halved and those who do manage to go spend less time there than earlier. Orphans in Uganda also face an increased risk of stunting and malnutrition.

(v) Threat to education system and social capital

AIDS threatens the educational system thus undermining the social capital of the country. In high-prevalence countries like Central African Republic, Côte d'lvoire and Zambia, it is eroding the supply of teachers and thus over crowding classes, which affects the quality of education.

(vi) Impact on cultivation and livestock

The effect on agricultural production can be serious. West Africa is a case in point. A study in Namibia by the Food and Agricultural Organisation (FAO) concluded that the impact on livestock was considerable, with a heavy gender bias: households headed by women and children generally lose their cattle, thus threatening the food security of the surviving members.

(vii) Increased absenteeism and lowered productivity at work

Companies in Africa are also experiencing the impact of HIV/AIDS on their balance sheets. Managers at one sugar estate in Kenya have noted increased absenteeism (8,000 days of work lost due to sickness between 1995 and 1997), lower productivity (a 50 per cent drop in the ratio of processed sugar recovered from raw cane between 1994 and 1997) and higher overtime costs for workers obliged to work longer hours to fill in for sick colleagues. Costs of social benefits related to HIV infection have increased sharply in the same company, due to funerals and health care costs.

(viii) Reduction in per capita income growth

Studies indicate that Africa's income growth per capita is being reduced by about 0.7 per cent per year because of HIV/AIDS. Had the HIV prevalence not reached 8.6 per cent in 1999, Africa's income per capita would have increased to 1.1 per cent per year - or nearly three times the growth rate of 0.4 per cent per year achieved in 1990-1997 (World Bank, 2000b). A country-specific econometric model of the South African economy suggests that overall GDP will be 17 per cent lower by 2010 than it would have been without AIDS and that average per capita income will be 7-10 per cent less because of AIDS (Lewis and Arndt, 2000).

Source: UNAIDS (2000a), pp. 26-36

Although some links have been well demonstrated in the above analysis, there are others for which the evidence is currently weak (Annexure 1). For the affected families and national policy-makers in many countries, however, the case is straightforward, AIDS is condemning millions to misery and poverty. Poverty includes not only low income and consumption but also low achievement in education, health, nutrition and overall human development. It includes powerlessness and vulnerability.

AIDS has left behind 13.2 million orphans - children who, before the age of 15, lost either their mother or both parents to AIDS. Many of these children have also died, but many more survive, not only in Africa (where 95 per cent currently live), but also in developing countries throughout Asia and the Americas. In African countries having, severe epidemics, AIDS is generating orphans so rapidly that family structures can no longer cope (UNAIDS, 2000a). In the absence of effective efforts to mitigate the effect of AIDS on this generation, whole societies will become dysfunctional, with serious consequences for human development and even basic security of mankind.

Funding in PRSPs and HIPC Documents

Even though there is increased awareness of the negative impact of HIV/AIDS on development, HIV/AIDS is only one of the problems that countries will address in their PRSPs and HIPC documents. There are many ministries, sectors and civil society groups trying to complete for attention and funding in PRSPs and HIPC documents. The case for HIV/AIDS must nevertheless is highly compelling. HIV/AIDS jeopardizes poverty reduction efforts, and by fighting AIDS poverty will also be tackled, so that money can be thus spent efficiently to reverse the epidemic and improve people's lives. Therefore, any effort to mainstream HIV/AIDS in the development agenda must be well expressed to ensure sponsors from multiple sectors and the highest levels of government. In order to be convincing, propagators of the use of debt relief savings for HIV/AIDS need to show how an effective national HIV/AIDS programme will contribute to the fight against poverty, while laying out the financial case for debt relief, including the cost to implement a far-reaching HIV/AIDS programme.

What Works Against HIV/AIDS?[1]

Effective responses to the HIV/AIDS epidemic would address the needs of each country, according to its requirement, depending on the status of the epidemic, the likely impact of a variety of cost-effective interventions in a given context, as well as the potential for large-scale programme planning, funding and implementation. The range of actions to fight the epidemic would include the development or strengthening of institutions for planning and coordination, multisectoral approaches to programme development and implementation, containment of new infections, affordable care for persons living with HIV/AIDS (PLWHAs), social support to minimise the impact of AIDS on families and orphans, as well as effective monitoring and evaluation of programme efforts. Country teams are likely to be more acceptable and effective advocates if their suggestions are based on experience of what works against HIV/AIDS, with clear outlines of the approaches to be taken in the national response to the epidemic and its consequences.

Although a lot remains to be understood about the evolution

of the epidemic and its consequences, much has been found out regarding effective interventions for HIV prevention, cost-effective care for persons who are already infected, and actions to reduce the impact on orphans, families and communities. When the first cases of AIDS were reported in the early 1980s, individuals and groups worked together to alert people to this dangerous new disease and the steps that could be taken to protect against it. Even before HIV was isolated, safer sex and reliable drug use guidelines had been developed based upon epidemiological evidence regarding patterns of transmission. However, providing people with information about how to guard against infection has proven to be insufficient? People require conducive environments that will reduce their susceptibility and vulnerability, and allow them to modify their behaviour based on their knowledge gained through information provision (UNAIDS, 2000a).

Conducive Environment for Effective Intervention Against AIDS

At the national level, political commitment at all levels is known to be essential for programme success. Multilevel interventions that seek to include a variety of partners in coordinated action are known to be more successful than those that work in isolation (UNAIDS, 1999, 2000a). Moreover, coordinated economic, political and social effort is required to reduce societal vulnerability, alongside programmes and interventions functioning at individual and community levels. Global experience has shown the following elements to be among those central to effective national HIV prevention efforts (Piot and Aggleton, 1998):

(i) *General awareness-raising activities* to provide information and counter negative reactions among the population as a whole.

(ii) *Focused persuasive action* to meet the needs of specially sensitive groups and communities, with steadily expanding coverage.

(iii) *Multisectoral and multilevel partnerships* to deliver programmes and services related to a range of contexts.

(iv) *Community ownership of programmes*, and persuading groups and individuals to contribute to national HIV prevention efforts.

(v) *Greater integration between prevention and care* to mitigate costs and levels of discrimination and stigmatization.

(vi) *Building societal resistance* to HIV transmission and reduce the vulnerability of particular individuals, groups and sections of society.

Guarding Against HIV Infection

There has been hardly any evidence on preventive interventions in the published literature. Merson *et al*. (2000) reviewed the success of projects and programmes in developing countries that aim at decreasing sexual transmission of HIV infection or transmission through injection drug use. They found that behavioural change measures are effective when targeted to populations at high risk, particularly female sex workers and their clients. There are hardly any studies evaluating harm reduction interventions in Injecting Drug Users (IDUs). Reaction on the effectiveness of voluntary counselling and testing prograrnmes was mixed, and results differed according to the population being studied. STI treatment resulted is being highly effective in reducing HIV/STI transmission, particularly in the earlier stages of the epidemic. Structural and environmental measures show great promise, although more evaluation is needed. Merson *et al*. concluded that:

- HIV prevention measures can be effective in changing risk behaviours and preventing transmission in low- and middle-income countries;
- when the suitable mix of interventions is applied, they can lead to substantial reductions in the prevalence of HIV at the national level; and
- additional research is needed to identify effective interventions, specially in men who have sex with men, youth, IDUs and HIV-infected persons.

In reality, countries will strike a pragmatic balance, based on the ability of prgramme implementation, the expected results of interventions, their political feasibility and the availability of financial resources. For all purposes, countries would need to consider measures aimed at reducing risk and those aimed at reducing vulnerability (Table 1).

TABLE - 1
INTERVENTIONS FOR PREVENTION OF HIV INFECTION

	Factors influencing transmission of HIV	*Interventions*
"Risk"-oriented strategies addressing immediate factors of transmission	• Sexual transmission	IEC for behaviour change School education Life skills Condoms (promotion of 100 per cent condom use among the most vulnerable, including CSWs and the military) Voluntary counselling and testing Counselling STI treatment
	• Blood transmission	Blood safety Universal precautions Safe injections/ needle exchange
	• Mother-to-child transmission	Prevention of mother-to-child transmission
"Vulnerability"—oriented strategies addressing underlying factors of transmission	• Sexual behaviour • Intravenous drug use • Cultural and religious factors • Poverty • Illiteracy • Discrimination	• Behaviour change education • Life skills and education for in-school and out-of-school youth • Harm reduction, • IEC for behaviour change • Community mobilization • Poverty reduction • Education
	• Migration	• Legislation • Human rights • Rural development, etc.

Resource Availability and Care and Support Packages

With millions infected and many more affected by HIV, the need of intervention has become urgent for improved access to affordable care, support and mitigation of the effect on individuals, communities and countries. Table 2 shows a summary of interventions to be considered for care, support and impact mitigation.

TABLE - 2
CARE AND SUPPORT PACKAGES, ACCORDING TO RESOURCE AVAILABILITY

Package	*Contents*
The essential package	• Voluntary HIV counselling and testing • Psychosocial support for HIV-positive people and their families • Palliative care and treatment for pneumonia, oral thrush, vaginal candidiasis and pulmonary tuberculosis • Prevention of infections with cotrimoxazole prophylaxis for symptomatic HIV-positive people • Official recognition and facilitation of community activities that reduce the impact of HIV infection
The intermediate package	**All of the above plus one or more of the following:** • Active case-finding (and treatment) of tuberculosis among HIV-positive people • Preventive therapy for tuberculosis for HIV-positive people • Systemic antifungals for systemic fungal infections (such as cryptococcosis) • Treatment of Kaposi sarcoma • Surgical treatment of cervical cancer • Treatment of extensive herpes with acyclovir • Funding for community activities that reduce the impact of HIV infection
The advanced package	**All of the above plus:** • Triple antiretroviral therapy • Diagnosis and treatment of opportunistic infections that are difficult to diagnose and/or expensive to treat, such as atypical mycobacterial infections, cytomegalovirus infection, multiresistant tuberculosis, toxoplasmosis and HIV-associated cancers • Specific public services that reduce the economic and social impacts of HIV, to supplement community efforts that reduce the impact of HIV infection

Source: UNAIDS (2000a), pp. 96-98.

Garnering Resources

Resources have to be modified for all aspects of the response to HIV/AIDS described above. For sub-Saharan Africa alone, mobilizing a wide range of interventions would require US$1.5-2.3 billion per year. Providing Highly Active Antiretroviral Therapy (HAART) would add another US$1.5-2.4 billion depending on the prices at which drugs would be available. These estimates are based on relatively conservative estimates of likely coverage that can be achieved by 2005 (World Bank, 2000c).

Country- specific estimates of the resource gaps will suggest the immediate use of additional resources. In Zambia, resources required for implementing the National HIV/AIDS Strategic Framework were to the time of US$558.6 million for 2001-2003. A total of US$25.5 million had been committed by October 2000, leaving a resource gap of US$382 million (Bail and Mwikisa, 2000).

Notes and Reference

1. A full review of interventions against HIV/AIDS is beyond the scope of this document. Readers who wish to explore these in detail are encouraged to examine the growing literature on prevention, care and impact mitigation, including Merson et al. (2000), UNAIDS (2000a), Ainsworth and Teokul (2000), Jha et al. (2000) and Hunter (2000).

Thirteen

Essential Aspects of HIV/AIDS Documents

The essential elements and aspects of AIDS need to be highlighted while presenting of PRSPs and HIPC documents. A comprehensive study of these aspects has been taken up in this chapter.

Meaning of PRSPs

Poverty Reduction Strategy Papers (PRSPs) are documents that are designed to specify the issues and approaches to poverty reduction in many developing countries, specially in the countries receiving debt relief under the enhanced HIPC. A successful poverty reduction strategy is expected to: (a) be prepared by the country; (b) focus on speedier and broad-based economic growth; (c) indicate a comprehensive understanding of poverty and its determinants; (d) assist in selecting public actions that have the highest poverty impact; and (e) set-up outcome indicators that are set and monitored using participatory processes.

Most low-income countries are not directly in a position to fully address each of the elements of a PRSP. Interim PRSPs (I-PRSPs) outline the process for producing full PRSPs, identify the gaps that need to be filled, and outline how this might be done (World Bank, 2000a). As of mid-January 2001, three countries had prepared PRSPs[1] while 29 had prepared I-PRSPs[2].

Debt Relief

The principal objective of debt relief for the heavily indebted poor countries (HIPCs) is to bring the country's debt burden to endurine levels, subject to satisfactory policy performance, so as to make sure that adjustment and reform efforts are not put at risk by continued high debt and debt service burdens. The process entails two key phases, the first culminating in the "decision point", and the second, in the "completion point". To reach the decision point a debtor country must have accomplished a three year period of satisfactory performance on the macroeconomic adjustment and reform programmes backed by the IMF and the World Bank. At the decision point, the Executive Boards of the IMF and the World Bank formally determine country's eligibility for debt relief and the international community commit to providing sufficient aid by completion point for the country to accomplish debt sustainability as assessed at the decision point. The HIPC initiative defines debt sustainability as 150 per cent of the level of export at net present value.

Most eligible countries will decrease their debt-to-export and debt-to-revenue ratios (net present value) between the decision and completion points. In short, under the intensified framework, the benefits of export and central government revenue will accrue fully to the country, thus permitting greater investment in poverty reduction strategies.[3] At decision point, the country usually takes advantages from about 30 per cent of the total amount of debt relief to be given. After passing the decision point, a country reaches the second phase and moves toward the completion point when the bulk of assistance under the Enhanced HIPC Initiative is delivered.

Interim assistance can be given between the decision point and the completion point, with any remaining assistance provided at the completion point. The term "floating completion point" refers to an agreement in which the timing of completion point is tied to the implementation of policies determined at decision point. Twenty two countries[4] have reached their decision point under the enhanced HIPC Initiative and one country (Uganda) reached its completion point under the original HIPC Initiative. These 22 countries have since been receiving relief that will total to some $34 billion over time.

Highlighting the Need for HIV/AIDS Control in Documents

While there has been no pre-set formula for drafting the Poverty Reduction Strategy Papers and HIPC debt relief documents, in-practice they have tended to follow a fairly standard format. Since teams in-charge of PRSP and HIPC in each country and their World Bank/IMF counterparts are likely to use this format, it is possible for those focusing on HIV/AIDS to prepare a set of materials that fit into the main sections of the poverty and debt relief documents.

Aspects of HIV/AIDS to be included in the documents

The PRSP and HIPC materials would cover at least four essential aspects:

(a) AIDS as a cause of poverty, and if possible to initiate a discussion of poverty and income inequalities as factors promoting conditions that make persons vulnerable to HIV infection and less able to cope with the after effects of being infected;

(b) the main strategies in the national AIDS plan as a theme of the overall national poverty reduction programme, justified and costed;

(c) medium-term goals and poverty monitoring indicators obtained from the national AIDS plan; and

(d) short-run actions for the successful functioning of the national AIDS plan, which could form agreements for debt relief

Cause and Effect Relationship of Poverty and AIDS

In this section, the general linkages between AIDS and poverty are mentioned as well as documented with specific examples from the country or from neighbouring countries where similar conditions prevail. Sources of data for this analysis include household surveys such as the Demographic and Health Surveys (DHS), special studies conducted under the national AIDS programme, macroeconomic models that factor in HIV/AIDS as a variable affecting labour productivity, health spending and budget analyses that are indicators of public expenditures on AIDS.

Impact indicators that help to represent the effects of AIDS on poverty include:

(a) decrease in per capita income growth rate,

(b) increase in number of AIDS orphans, their corresponding poorer nutrition and halving of education,

(c) reductions in productivity and cash income in households with an AIDS death, and
(d) increased medical expenditure.

While initiating the design of a PRSP or preparing an interim PRSP for the purpose of obtaining debt relief, it is important for HIV/AIDS decision-makers to be able to present an overview of the relationship between HIV/AIDS and poverty. It will help as an advocacy tool to make a case for HIV/AIDS and to prepare the analytical rationale for choosing the most suitable and cost-effective interventions in a context of poverty reduction.

Basic analysis would include an estimation of the current situation, its seriousness as well as the threat it poses to the future. These topics could be covered through a presentation of the evolution of the HIV epidemic countrywide and a projection of the development of the epidemic if the reaction is not accelerated. The analysis of the HIV prevalence between regions of different economic development and among different vulnerable groups will help demarcate high-prevalence areas and link them with behaviours as well as economic exchange patterns (HIV epidemic mapping). A disaggregated analysis of the HIV prevalence by gender and age group is useful, to prove that young girls are among the groups most threatened by HIV. Sensitive factors can also be discussed using both quantitative and qualitative information. This analysis would attempt to simplify how some key socioeconomic determinants may affect the spread of HIV and what is the hard evidence available on this issue. Finally a quick analysis of the response can be conducted including an assessment of the proportion of cities covered by a programme for commercial sex workers, the proportion of roads covered by a programme for truck drivers, etc.

AIDS Plan and Poverty Reduction Strategies

These would comprise four to six well-defined strategies from the country's plan for an enhanced response for prevention, care, support and impact mitigation, based on expected effect, cost-effectiveness and feasibility, with cost estimates. Even if the national AIDS plan consists of many more strategies, it will probably be important to select the most important ones, since the PRSP is quite a brief document. Country teams might also choose to state the incremental resources needed for recurrent line items, such as for personnel, transportation, supplies and materials. In a few well-written Poverty Reduction Strategies to date in high HIV prevalence countries, AIDS is presented in the PRSP as requiring a strategic response that cuts across the traditional sectors, covering health, education, defence, transport, youth, communications and others. Meaning thereby that the main lines of the national AIDS plan are first presented as a "supra-sectoral" or "cross-cutting" concern, and this is then reinforced in the paragraphs devoted to the main poverty-fighting sectors, where AIDS again appears as a threat requiring special actions from each sector agency and from civil society groups and donors focusing on the sector. The Malawi PRSP is a useful example of this approach Table 1.

TABLE 1

SELECTED EXAMPLES OF PRSPS, AND THEIR HIV/AIDS CONTENTS*

Country	*Country-specific analysis of the AIDS-poverty complex*	*Main strategies from the national AIDS plan*	*Medium-term goals and poverty monitoring indicators*	*Short-run actions*
Cameroon (Interim PRSP, August, 2000)	HIV/AIDS not mentioned under "determinants of poverty".	Subsumed under health sector: "the principal and most urgent concern is the spread of HIV/AIDS". Specific actions to slow the progression: IEC, VCT, and blood safety. Brief mention under "Urban Poverty", focusing on commercial sex workers. Emphasis on education campaigns.	"Rate of HIV/AIDS incidence".	Set up HIV/AIDS information and awareness campaigns in public and private media.

(Contd.)

(Contd.)

Country	*Country-specific analysis of the AIDS-poverty complex*	*Main strategies from the national AIDS plan*	*Medium-term goals and poverty monitoring indicators*	*Short-run actions*
Malawi (Interim PRSP, August 2000)	Included as part of "Super-Sectoral Analysis", with references to country-specific statistics on seropreva-lence. There are explicit notes on the effects on growth, poverty, productivity and savings. Orphans and families get specific attention. Reference to the National Strategic Framework for HIV/AIDS and the Resource Mobilization Round Table of March 2000.	Under "strategies and measures:. Mainstream HIV/AIDS into all sectors and improve orphan care. Intensify efforts on primary prevention. Integrate AIDS and tuberculosis control programmes. Strengthen AIDS Secretariat.	Not specified.	Not specified.
Uganda (PRSP-Poverty Eradication Action Plan, March 2000)	Under "improving health of the people". There are notes on prevalence rates, effects on life expectancy, as well as a brief acknowledgement of interactions among AIDS, cultural factors and poverty.	Expenditures for service delivery to be included in health and other sectors. Note: Based on its National Strategic Framework, Uganda subsequently revised its Poverty Eradication Action Plan to include AIDS in each of the four goals. The National Strategic Framework emphasizes prevention, impact mitigation and capacity building.	25% decline in HIV preva-lence. Short-run actions	Not specified.

* A convenience sample of three countries, for illustration. Source: World Bank Website on PRSPs.
http://www.world bank. org/prsp/. Accessed on 31 January 2001.

Formulating Medium-term Goals and Targets

The medium term goals also need to be selective, as only a few AIDS strategies are likely to be listed in the PRSP. Ideally, these goals and indicators will have been developed with technical knowhow, and negotiated among stakeholders as part of the AIDS national planning process. In many instances this will not have happened, either because the national AIDS plan is not complete or because goal/target setting was not implemented as part of the national planning process. Since the medium term covers five years or more into the future, the goals would relate to results of the national AIDS response - outcomes ideally, or at least major achievements of the AIDS programme. Each country team will need to formulate medium-term goals and targets that are right for national circumstances. Uganda has specified a 25 per cent decline in HIV prevalence as its medium-term goal. A convenience sample of three countries, (Cameroon, Malawai and Uganda) was taken to analyse the strategies from the National AIDS Plan, the Medium-term goals and Poverty monitoring indicators as shown in Table 2.

TABLE - 2
MEASURES TO REACH THE FLOATING COMPLETION POINT UNDER THE HIPC INITIATIVE

Country	*Country-specific analysis of the AIDS-poverty complex*	*Main strategies from the national AIDS plan*	*Medium-term goals and poverty monitoring indicators*	*Short-run indicators with "conditions for debt relief*
Cameroon **Malawi Uganda**	Under "overall policy framework". Based on interim PRSP.	Included explicitly. Covers coordination mechanisms, overall goal, interventions and coverage indicators. Mentions line ministries involved.	Limit infection rate to below 10%. US$8.9 million over 3 years from HIPC proceeds for HIV/AIDS	Prioritize HIV/AIDS in overall agenda. Curb infection rates among population, with increased use of condoms among port workers, truckers, soldiers and commercial sex workers.

(Contd.)

(Contd.)

(1)	(2)	(3)	(4)	(5)
Malawi	Impact on life expectancy. Large number of orphans. Potential to reduce economic growth, not country-specific.	Proposed institutional framework: make National AIDS Control Programme secretariat autonomous, outside the control of any specific sectors. Summary of interventions for prevention, care and impact mitigation.	Not explicit. "Slowing the spread of AIDS" is a floating completion point trigger.	Policy areas to be monitored include a fully staffed, functional and autonomous National AIDS Control Secretariat.
Uganda	Specific notes in the Second Decision Point Document, including prevalence, life expectancy and Human Development Index. The poor are more likely to include widows, orphans and those living with HIV/AIDS.	Poverty Reduction Strategy for 1990/2000-2001/2002. Establishment of functional coordination mechanisms, at the central and district levels, for the national multisectoral response to HIV/AIDS. Expanded outreach of education for behaviour change.	Not specified.	Government established a Poverty Action Fund, under which programmes are outcome-oriented. Outcomes are reviewed on a quarterly basis with donors and representatives of civil society.

Source: World Bank Website on HIPC, http://www.world bank.org/hipc/country-cases/country-cases.html. Accessed on 31 January 2001.

Ideal Features of Short-run Actions Specified in Debt Relief Documents

Selectivity is also needed here. The Short-run actions are the agreed steps for decision and completion points, and that could be inserted into the matrix in the HIPC document. Ideally, they would have the features outlined below.

(a) The actions should be evolved from and closely connected to the key strategies in the national AIDS plan, spelled out earlier in the PRSP/HIPC document — in this sense, they should be seen as "sentinel" actions that specify whether the AIDS plan is being successfully implemented.

(b) The actions should be comparatively easy to measure. Since programme implementation will be monitored closely under HTC by government, civil society, and international agencies, it is important to set up an effective monitoring system that can generate results quickly.

(c) The actions should be carefully chosen to match the schedule for HIPC, especially the trigger points for entering debt relief (decision point), and intermediate and final (completion) debt forgiveness points.

(d) The actions should be well understood and acknowledged by the political figures and programme managers who will be answerable for implementing this series of actions.

Fortunately, there are a variety of indicators for monitoring and assessing the progress in implementing national AIDS programme strategies, which have already been initiated, and for which corresponding data collection and analysis methods are fairly well established. The UNAIDS Guide to Monitoring and Evaluation (UNAIDS, 2000c) is a handy abridgement of these indicators, an abbreviated set of which is presented in Annexure 2. At country level, too, national specialists on HIV/AIDS and international staff serving on the "technical working groups" of the United Nations Theme Groups on HIV/AIDS can help to select and justify the best performance targets for the period of HIPC debt relief.

PRSPs and their HIV Contents

Most I-PRSPs in sub-Saharan Africa have included HIV/AIDS as an issue to be tackled (Table 3). Yet the connection between HIV/AIDS and poverty has rarely been examined and the strategies do not appear very well layed out. In particular the vision of how the country will evolve a response to mitigate the negative effect of HIV/AIDS on human capital and economic growth has not been defined clearly in any of the PRSPs. However, Uganda is reshaping its strategy to better mainstream the issue of HIV/AIDS within its vision of poverty reduction.

Pre-requisites of the HIPC Initiative

On account of the policy dialogue surrounding debt relief, some countries have committed to increasing their efforts towards reducing the HIV/AIDS epidemic. The commitment has sometimes resulted into some conditionalities for the country to reach the completion point at which the major part of debt relief will be granted. Most of these conditionalities are process-related, yet some countries have committed to bringing about a real behaviour change as in Cameroon, where increased condom use among men in uniform, truck drivers and commercial sex workers was included as a pre-requisite.

The Cameroonian Experience and Strategy for Successful Implementation

The Cameroonian experience devotes several elements of a successful effort to integrate HIV/AIDS into an interim PRSP and a debt relief agreement.

During the last few years, the pace of activities had slowed down in Cameroon's response to HIV/AIDS. Though the National AIDS Control Programme administered a number of projects that were considered successful. The overall response was small-scale, divided and incomplete, however. At the same time the epidemic continued to spread, with more than 540,000 Cameroonians infected with HIV by the end of 1999 - a prevalence rate of 7.7 per cent among adults. (UNAIDS, 2000a). The debt relief discussions and the drafting of the Interim PRSP, which started in mid 2000 helped to bring about a more vigorous response to HIV/AIDS.

The I-PRSP was prepared during April-August 2000 with broad input from government and civil society, including NGOs and religious leaders, and published in September 2000. It highlighted HIV/AIDS of being responsible in worsening the country's poverty and as a grave threat to overall social and economic development. Similarly, at the initial stages of the debt negotiations, the government and World Bank officials identified AIDS as one of the most important areas that could benefit from additional resources from debt relief. This in turn encouraged the Government of Cameroon to speed up the development of a nationwide plan to contain the epidemic. An HIV/AIDS strategic planning process already under way in Cameroon was expedited to coincide with the debt negotiations. Thereafter the AIDS strategic plan became a precondition for finalizing the debt relief agreement, and the plan was also required to specify the priority actions in AIDS prevention and care that could be funded with debt relief savings.

As a results, the government finalized a comprehensive national HIV/AIDS strategic plan for 2001-2003, in collaboration with UNAIDS and other partners. It was launched by the Prime Minister of Cameroon in September 2000. The plan consisted of a set of highly concentrated emergency actions costing about US$9 million over three years, to be funded by the government using debt relief savings:

(a) initiating behaviour change in young people aged 15-24 through information, education and communication at the national and local levels,

(b) making voluntary testing and counselling widely available all over the country and preventing HIV transmission from pregnant women to their babies, and

(c) backing up a 100 per cent condom use campaign including free provision of condoms among key vulnerable groups: truckers, plantation workers, university students, military, police, workers in the customs service, prisoners, prison wardens and commercial sex workers.

Simultaneous to the debt relief process, the government and World Bank together prepared a major project, the Multisectoral Programme to Fight against HIV/AIDS, to be funded with a combination of a US$50 million World Bank credit (soft loan, partial grant) and national funding from debt relief savings. The World Bank credit was passed in December 2000, and the project was officially launched in February 2001. To administer the implementation of the ambitious national AIDS plan and the Bank-funded project, the government decided to establish a new Central Technical Group with a wide spectrum of skills in managing local and sectoral AIDS responses, communications, and monitoring and evaluation. The Cameroonian experience denotes the importance of high-level political commitment, a multisectoral approach, and a parallel focus on actions that are likely to have a significant impact on the epidemic. PRSP, HIPC, national AIDS planning, and a focus on implementation are closely interconnected.

Lessons Learnt

(a) the requirement for analysts working on HIV/AIDS to develop short, simple and clear advocacy materials for political decision-makers, including success stories from other countries,

(b) the heed of developing a vision of a national-scale response, with accurate estimates of the level of effort required to curtail the epidemic,

(c) the need to provide decision-makers with politically suitable options and visible short-run gains in fighting AIDS, using debt relief savings, and

(d) the importance of a planning process for PRSP and HIPC that is both participatory and substantive, maintaining a focus on practical and suitable actions that can be carried out to address the HIV/AIDS epidemic.

Specifying Amount of Savings on AIDS Programme

In increasing numbers of the HIPC debt relief documents, the budgetary savings from debt relief are clearly calculated for a number of years to come. There is thus a chance in the HIPC document to specify or demarcate how much of the savings (either as a percentage of the actual savings, or in absolute dollar terms) will be assigned to the national AIDS programme. If so, the teams working on HIV/AIDS in the HIPC process have an opportunity to lobby for a sizeable allocation to the national AIDS programme. This can be explained both on the basis of the estimated cost of a large-scale national response to the epidemic, and by demonstrating how important the fight against AIDS is in the overall effort to reduce poverty and promote economic and social development.

In high-prevalence countries, a minimum of US$1.50-2.00 per capita is required for a strong national AIDS programme which amounts to 15-20 million annually in a country with 10 million inhabitants. If one-quarter or one-half of these costs can be met through debt relief, with the balance being met from external development partners, this would constitute an important financial and political investment by the government.

As HIV/AIDS is cross-cutting issue that goes beyond any individual sector, a supra-sectoral budgeting/allocation is recommended. Earmarking debt relief savings for HIV/AIDS could itself be one of the HIPC prerequisites monitored for successful completion of the debt relief process. For example, "during the period from 2001-2003, the government will spend US$xx million of debt relief savings on its national AIDS programme".

Assigning Funds to Local Group Initiatives

A number of HIPC countries, recommend that a major portion of the debt relief savings assigned to AIDS - and probably, the entire budget to support the national AIDS plan - is channelled speedily and efficiently to local initiatives. These include local government units, local NGOs, and community organisations that are engaged in prevention, care and support activities. In this background the HIPC process can be a chance to develop and set up effective mechanisms for moving financial and technical resources to local groups implementing AIDS control activities. This can be carried out through a number of means that might be specified and monitored as part of national compliance with the conditions for debt relief, like the setting up a special "Poverty Action Fund" that receives the debt relief savings and uses them exclusively for local initiatives. These Poverty Action Funds are in part an accounting system, but when combined with resource transfer features, such as matching grants for local government bodies and NGOs, they can be a method of getting the resources out to the frontlines.

In Uganda, the Poverty Action Fund (PAF) includes the highest-priority expenditures from the viewpoint of poverty eradication. The inclusion of a particular sector or programme for funding from the Uganda PAF depends on high economic and/or social returns to the expenditure, by pro-poor functioning and by the priority accorded to such programmes by the poor themselves, as demonstrated by prior participatory work. Managers of the Malawi Social Action Fund (MASAF) in collaboration with the UNAIDS Secretariat and the World Bank , are finding out options to channel funds to communities for a more speedier implementation of activities to minimise the impact of AIDS. Direct funding of community-based activities is an important feature of the Africa Multicountry AIDS Programme that was initiated by the World Bank in 2000 (World Bank, 2000b). In the same way, if all or part of the debt relief savings were put in a national social development fund or micro-projects fund with a clear HIV/AIDS component, this could be another method to ensure that the savings reach local public and/or private institutions (e.g. youth clubs, women's groups, NGOs assisting commercial sex workers, village AIDS committees). The establishment of these kinds of initiatives for transferring debt relief savings to local groups could be clearly laid out in the HIPC documents as completion point objectives.

Accountability of Funds Released through HIPC

The HIPC process gives an opportunity to create strong mechanisms for accountability for uses of financial resources and for results. In a number of countries, civil society groups and international donors are demanding procedures that make the use of debt relief savings and donor funds more transparent and linked to accountable programme results. One way was to establish mixed bodies (composed of representatives of government, civil society, and donor agencies) to monitor progress and use of funds in parts or all of the national AIDS programme. This is the method used in Uganda, where quarterly reviews are carried out with representation from donors and civil society.

In Malawi, the expenditure monitoring methods for HIPC resources include public reporting of expenditures. As far as possible, assessments of output, outcome and impact should be undertaken to measure the benefits of inputs through various financing mechanisms. Distribution of funds could be accompanied by the collection of household and community-level data as part of a baseline assessment. This would make easy the evaluation of a funding mechanisms as well as the projects financed through the funding mechanism (Ram, 2000).

How to get the HIV/AIDS Issues into PRSP/Debt. Relief Agenda

After focusing on the reasons why HIV/AIDS belongs to PRSP and HIPC agenda and on what to include in the agreements in this section we shall focus on the How of getting the HIV/AIDS issues into the PRSP/Debt. Relief Agenda. The above can be achieved by:

(a) Building Coalitions, and
(b) Strengthening Capacity

Building Coalitions of Diverse Groups

To build coalitions, it is necessary that the diverse groups that are already committed to fighting the HIV epidemic collect together, and bring in others who are not yet fully convinced. These could include parts of government including the national AIDS secretariat or coordinating body, the national AIDS council or inter-ministerial committee, AIDS units in some ministries, civil society groups that are already functioning and often have one or several national umbrella organisations, associations of people living with HIV/AIDS and a wide range of multilateral, bilateral, and international nongovernmental agencies. To back the PRSP and HIPC process, these numerous individuals and institutions can be engaged as members of task forces, inter-agency working groups, etc., led by government and other national actors. So as to influence the process and content of the PRSP and debt relief agreements, the HIV/AIDS "coalition" must not only express a strong case for including HIV/AIDS on "technical" grounds, but also be closely engaged with those responsible for overall preparation and negotiation of the PRSP/HIPC instruments. These include senior officials of the Ministry of Finance and/or national economics and planning agency, and technical officers from the World Bank and International Monetary Fund. It will be also useful to have an inter-agency committee or technical working group supporting the Ministry of Finance team, on which certain persons from the HIV/AIDS coalition can serve. The ministries involved include those of education, social development, youth, defence, agriculture and transport.

Focusing national media attention on AIDS as a poverty issue and a threat to development can also be important in influencing national policy on AIDS in the PRSP and debt relief initiatives. The Uganda AIDS Commission led a process that was both inclusive and participatory, the accomplishment of which provided a basis for incorporating AIDS into all the goals of the country's Poverty Eradication Action Plan.

The PRSP/HIPC initiative can also be an opportunity to build greater technical capacity in-country to deal with a multitude of analytical and managerial challenges inherent in mounting and sustaining a strong national AIDS programme. As experienced from the above, effective inclusion of HIV/AIDS in the PRSP and HIPC needs among other — skills in analysing the impact of AIDS on poverty, programme priority setting and costing, negotiation, and monitoring and evaluation. For each of these areas, a few capable individuals must be located in key institutions, including the national AIDS secretariat, the Ministry of Finance, and National NGO umbrella organisations and associations of people living with HIV/AIDS.

Minimum Capacity Building

The PRSP/HIPC initiative requires that members of the AIDS "coalition" in the country should develop, fund and implement an environment for minimum capacity building to support the process. Carrying out this capacity building could also be one of the related objectives under PRSP and debt relief, and could be explicitly financed and monitored as part of HIPC. Such a minimum scheme should specify the required skills and the institutions which include these skills. The scheme of things resembles the following parameters:

(a) *National AIDS Secretariat:* one planner and one economist trained in programming, priority setting, costing, and monitoring/evaluation.

(b) *Ministry of Finance:* one economist attached to PRSP/HIPC who can assemble data on the poverty-AIDS linkage and clarify AIDS commitments under debt relief.

(c) *Poverty Action Fund and/or AIDS portfolio within the national social development fund:* 2-3 person management teams trained to sustain both the programmatic and financial dimensions of a major transfer of resources to local AIDS initiatives.

(d) *The umbrella NGO organisation and PLWHA association:* at least one person in each who can help in clarifying key commitments on AIDS under debt relief and assist in monitoring compliance with AIDS conditions under HIPC.

Ways of Optimizing the use of Debt Relief Funds

In many countries while accessing debt relief, the HIV/AIDS programme managers and decision-makers have the opportunity to claim more funding for HIV/AIDS in a context of the development of poverty reduction strategies. Debt relief does not only provide the chance of obtaining fresh resources in the fight against HIV, it also gives the opportunity to place HIV/AIDS at the centre of the development and aid agenda and to discuss country issues linked to policy development and budgeting. Despite of being provided with external resources through various initiatives, many HIV/AIDS programmes in poor countries have not yet reached a point that will influence the pattern of the epidemic. Increases in internal revenue available for the social sectors may provide the opportunity to reach that scale by:

(i) placing HIV/AIDS within the purview of budgetary discussions, and breaking the cycle of donor-driven programme design and financing;

(ii) institutionalizing the response to HIV/AIDS in all activities of the government, utilizing the new fiscal space to provide additional resources to each sector for this specific purpose;

(iii) transforming dispersed activities into sustained programmes, thus freeing the country from extreme dependence on donors for key inputs (for example, financing drugs for tuberculosis control or condoms for the military) and ensuring a constant supply of such commodities; and

(iv) addressing broader issues not always directly linked to HIV/AIDS but often strongly affecting the reaction and contributing to dysfunction in the sectors through staff friction, poor remuneration and paucity of funds for recurrent expenditures.

Country officials and their partners who are policy-makers and managers have a reason to think objectively about how different sources of funding can complement each other rather than compete to fund the same programmes. Debt relief funds may be used wisely so as to develop the capacity to exert influence and absorb further available external funding. In Mali, for example, while the health sector benefits from a large externally funded sector investment programme, HIPC funds are likely to be utilized to strengthen the implementation capacity by financing basic training as well as contracting of staff and giving incentives for them to deliver essential public health interventions.

The pattern followed by poor countries to date in integrating HIV/AIDS in poverty strategies and debt relief has been mixed. Though there have been some notable successes, but also a number of failures and missed opportunities. UNAIDS and its partners stand ready to help countries affected by the HIV epidemic to get hold more fully the current and future opportunities to bring HIV/AIDS to the forefront of the analysis and national actions to combat poverty and gain maximum benefits from debt relief.

Annexure 1
Links Between HIV/AIDS and Poverty

AIDS Induces or worsens poverty

The link between AIDS and poverty are examined at the levels of the individual, the household and the national economy. Once infected, the individual expenses direct catastrophic costs in terms of health and social care, plus indirect costs in terms of lost productivity. Most likely, the household is expected to experience reduced income. Business productivity is most likely to decline, due to lost productivity, high absenteeism, increased payments for treatment and funerals, as well as increased costs of training and retraining of replacements for dead workers. Figures A1 and A2 indicate the pathways from HIV infection to increased poverty.

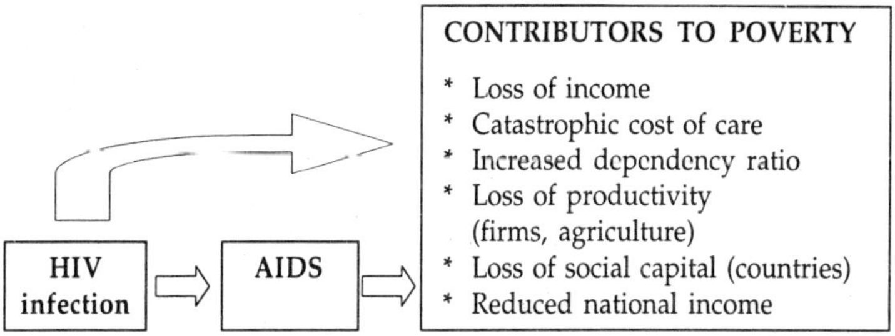

FIG. A1: HIV/AIDS INDUCES AND DEEPENS POVERTY

AIDS as an Outcome of Income Inequalities and Poverty

The general pathways by which poverty and income inequalities increase an individual's chances of becoming infected with HIV are perhaps indirect. Increased sensitivity to HIV infection is necessary because it increases the chances of transmitting or becoming infected with HIV. Thus poverty may reduce an individual's ability or willingness to avoid becoming infected. For instance, income poverty may lead people to engage in high-risk income-generating activities such as commercial sex work. Commercial sex workers may indulge in sex without condoms in exchange of higher fees. Poverty often results in lower education, which may in turn be associated with lower awareness of effective measures to prevent HIV infection.

Figure A2 and Box A1 indicate the route through which poverty leads to increased risks of HIV infection. Till today, there is not enough systematic evidence to support an assertion that poverty causes AIDS. While it is most likely that some of the features of poverty (e.g. lower educational level, fewer livelihood choices, lower capacity to negotiate safe sex) also increase the chances of being infected with HIV, it would not be fully correct to see HIV purely as a "disease of the poor". Many groups and individuals at high risk of being infected with HIV in Africa (urban elite who purchase sex, travelling businessmen who have casual sex, officers in the armed forces) are not among the poor. At this stage of the epidemic, HIV/AIDS transcends all household economic boundaries. For prevention, it is understood from the literature available that in the short to medium term, the high-impact interventions are those that mitigate the risk of transmitting the virus or the risk of becoming infected.

Risk factors are those elements that increase directly the chances that an individual will become infected with HIV as a carrier. Interventions focusing on vulnerability reduction are structural or more intensive development challenges. They could have indirect effects on the dynamics of the epidemic. Clearly there needs to be a redressal for medium- to long-term success against HIV/AIDS. However, the after effects of the epidemic are such that any laxity to act on risk reduction would result in a substantially larger number of infected persons, further limiting the gains from structural interventions against vulnerability.

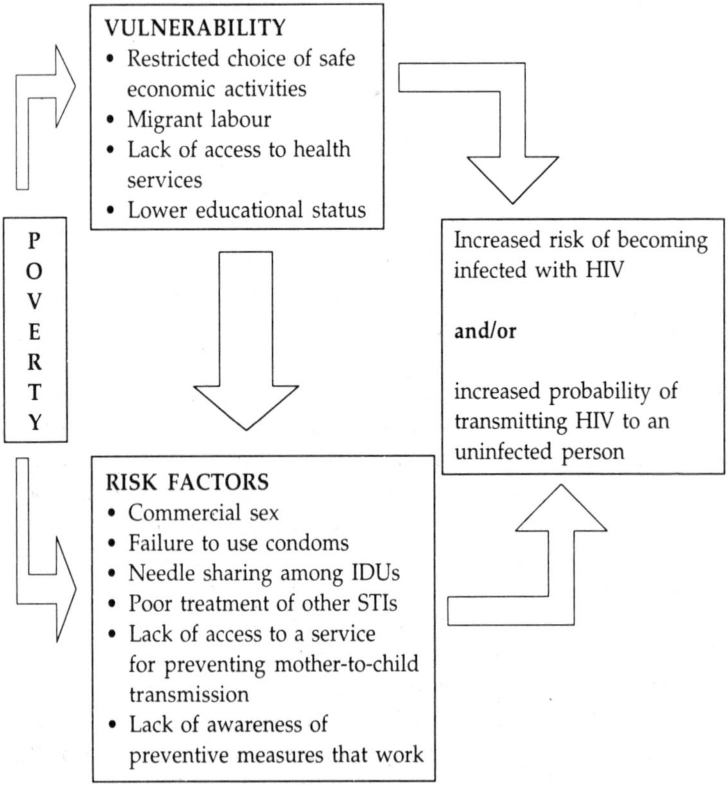

FIG A2: POVERTY INCREASES THE LIKELIHOOD OF HIV INFECTION AND AIDS

Plausible Pathways though which Poverty Leads to Increased Risks for HIV Infection

During the initial years of the HIV/AIDS epidemic, persons of higher socioeconomic status were more likely than others to become infected with HIV. As HIV/AIDS becomes common in most African countries, the positive correlation between socio-economic status and HIV infection could be expected to disappear. The proof to this effect are mixed, as related in the following paragraphs. Among the issues requiring attention is the combined effect of poverty and income inequalities in social relationships including sex, patterns of vulnerability and risky behaviour in relation to HIV infection.

Indicators of Correlation between socio-economic status and AIDS

(i) UNAIDS analysed the results of research carried out among 15-19-year olds in 17 African and four Latin American countries. A pattern, of vulnerability, seen in both sexes, was that more educated individuals were generally more likely to have casual partners (UNAIDS, 2000a). The results also showed that the best-educated people in the hardest-hit countries in Africa may be moving towards less risky behaviour (UNAIDS, 2000a). Although it is yet early to tell, this pattern seems like that in Brazil, where there has been a change in socioeconomic distribution of AIDS cases: in the early 1980s, three fourths of those newly diagnosed with AIDS had a secondary or university education; by the early 1990s this share had fallen to one-third (Parker, 1998).

(ii) Poverty and illiteracy might be more likely to raise the chances of infection with sexually transmitted diseases, including HIV/AIDS, since people with low incomes may be less capable than those with higher incomes to afford condoms or STI treatment and those with little education may have less access to information about the harms caused by high-risk behaviour of may be less able to decipher prevention messages. This justifies the reason why, for most STIs, the poor and uneducated have higher infection rates (Lacey et al., 1997). It also appears to be the case for the spread of HIV in industrialized countries (Cowan *et al.*, 1994; Krueger *et al.*, 1990; McCoy *et al.*, 1996).

(iii) During the first decade of the HIV/AIDS epidemic in Africa, HIV infections followed a different pattern. A number of studies therefore showed a positive correlation between HIV infection and socioeconomic status, measured by schooling, income or occupation (Ainsworth and Semali, 1998). While examining data from demographic and health surveys carried out during the early 1990s and surveys of sexual behaviour sponsored by the WHO Global Programme on AIDS (GPA) conducted in 1989-1991 we see that the chances of having a non-regular or commercial sexual partner rise with education level, potentially increasing exposure to contracting STIs, including HIV (Filmer 1998; Deheneffe *et al.*, 1998). The demand for commercial sex and/or the potential to support multiple partners would rise with income. Also, persons with higher education and higher incomes have more disposable cash and are more likely to travel - thus having more opportunities for casual sex.

(iv) Total income does not alone predict trends in HIV prevalence: intracountry social and cultural factors play important roles in the dynamics of the epidemic. While well-meaning statements like "poverty causes" AIDS may appear implicitly pro-poor, they may actually hamper condom promotion and other on the-around prevention efforts (Halperin, 2000).

Annexure 2
INDICATORS

1. Overview of indicators by programme areas, tools for measurement, and priority for different epidemic states*

(C=Core indicator; A=Additional indicator)

Note: Country teams are encouraged to refer to the full text for definitions and to be highly selective in their use of indicators.

Programme area indicator	*Priority Generalized epidemic*	*Priority Concentrated/ low-level*
Policy		
1. Spending on HIV prevention	C	C
Condom availability and quality		
1. Condoms available, nationwide	C	C
2. Condoms available, retail	C	A
Stigma and discrimination		
1. Accepting attitudes toward HIV+ people	C	C
2. Employers not discriminating	C	C
Knowledge		
1. Knowledge of HIV prevention	C	C
Voluntary counselling and testing		
1. People who requested test and received results	C	A
2. Districts with VCT services	C	
3. VCT centres with minimum conditions	C	A
4. Quality of VCT laboratories	A	A
Mother-to-child transmission		
1. Pregnant women counselled and tested	C	
2. Antenatal clinics offering and referring for antenatal care	C	
3. Quality HIV counselling for pregnant women	A	
4. Provision of antiretroviral therapy	A	
Sexual negotiation and attitudes		
1. Women's ability to negotiate safe sex	A	
Sexual behaviour		
1. Higher-risk sex in the last year	C	C
2. Condom use at last higher-risk sex	C	C
3. Commercial sex in last year	A	C
4. Condom use by clients at last paid sex	A	C
5. Condom use by sex workers with last client	A	A

* Part of the Behavioural surveillance surveys (BSS): Guidelines for repeated behavioural surveys in population groups at risk for HIV

2. Overview of indicators by programme areas, tools for measurement, and priority for different epidemic states*

(C=Core indicator; A=Additional indicator)

Note: Country teams are encouraged to refer to the full text for definitions and to be highly selective in their use of indicators.

Programme area indicator	*Priority Generalized epidemic*	*Priority Concentrated/ low-level*
Young people's sexual behaviour		
1. Median age at first sex	C	
2. Young people having premarital sex	C	A
3. Condom use at last premarital sex	C	A
4. Young people with multiple partners	C	A
5. Condom use at last higher-risk sex	C	A
6. Condom use at first sex	A	A
7. Age-mixing in sexual relationships	A	
Injecting drug use		
1. Injecting drug users sharing equipment		C
2. Injecting drug users never sharing equipment		C
3. Drug injectors using condom at last sex		A
Blood safety/nosocomial transmission		
1. Screening of blood units for transfusion	C	C
2. Reduction of blood transfusions	A	A
3. Districts/regions with blood bank	C	C
4. Accidental transmission in health care settings	A	
STI care and prevention		
1. Appropriate diagnosis and treatment of STI	C	C
2. Advice on prevention and HIV testing	C	C
3. Drug supply at STI care services	C	A
4. Treatment seeking for STI	A	C
Care and support		
1. Medical personnel trained in AIDS	A	A
2. Health facilities with capacity to deliver care	C	
3. Health facilities with drugs in stock	A	
4. Households helped with care of young adults	C	
5. Households helped with care of orphans	A	
Health and social impact		
1. HIV prevalence among pregnant women	C	C
2. Syphilis prevalence among pregnant women	C	C
3. HIV prevalence in sub-populations at risk	A	C
4. Prevalence of orphanhood	C	
5. Schooling of orphans	A	

* Part of the Behavioural surveillance surveys (BSS): Guidelines for repeated behavioural surveys in population groups at risk for HIV.

Annexure 3

SELECTED WEBSITES ON AIDS, POVERTY AND DEBT RELIEF

http://www.unaids.org/publications/documents/index.html
http://www.worldbank.org/hipc/
http://www.worldbank.org/aids-econ/
http://www.worldbank.org/poverty/
http://www.oxfam.org/advocacy/human_f.htm
http://www.dfid.gov.uk/public/what/strategy_papers/target_strategy.html
http://www.usaid.gov/pop_health/aids/index.html
http://www.j2000.usa.org

References

Ainsworth, M., Semali, 1. 1998. "Who is most likely to die of AIDS? Socioeconomic correlates of adult deaths in Kagera Region, Tanzania." In Ainsworth, M., Fransen, L, Over, M. (Eds). *Confronting AIDS: Evidence from the developing world*. Selected background papers for the World Bank Policy Research Report, *Confronting AIDS: Public priorities in a global epidemic*. European Commission, Brussels, pp. 95-109.

Ainsworth, M., Teokul, W. 2000. "Breaking the silence: setting realistic priorities for AIDS control in less-developed countries." *The Lancet*. 356:35-40.

Bail, R., Mwikisa, C. *Costing the Zambia National HIV/AIDS Strategic Framework 2001-2003*. Unpublished manuscript, October 2000, pp. 8-10.

Cowan, D. Brundage, J., Pomerantz, R. 1994. "The incidence of HIV infection among men in the United States". *AIDS* 8 (4): 505-11.

Deheneffe, J., Carael, M., Noumbissi, A. 1998. Socioeconomic Determinants of Sexual Behaviour and Condom Use". In Ainsworth, M., Fransen, L, Over, M. (Eds). *Confronting AIDS: Evidence from the developing world*. Selected background papers for the World Bank Policy Research Report, *Confronting AIDS: Public Priorities in a global epidemic*. European Commission, Brussels, pp. 131-46.

Filmer, D. 1998. "The Socioeconomic Correlates of Sexual Behaviour: A Summary of Results from an Analysis of DHS Data". In Ainsworth, M., Fransen, L, Over, M. (Eds). *Confronting AIDS: Evidence from the developing world*. Selected background papers for the World Bank Policy Research Report, *Confronting AIDS: Public Priorities in a global epidemic*. European Commission, Brussels, pp. 111-30.

Halperin, D. 2000. "Is Poverty the Root Cause of African AIDS? The 'Answer' May Be More Complex Than Commonly Thought". *Global AIDS Link*, Global Health Council, 65:9.

Hunter, S. *National Systems and Strategies for Provision of Care to HIV/AIDS Affected Adults and Children*. A discussion paper presented at the UNAIDS Workshop on the Role of Debt Relief in Financing National HIV/AIDS Programmes. Lilongwe, Malawi. November, 2000. Unpublished manuscript, pp. 1-2.

Jha, P., Nagelkerke, N., Ngugi, E., Rao, J., Willbond, B., Moses, S., Plummer, F. 2000. "Interventions to Reduce HIV Transmission in Developing Countries: The Lessons of Two Decades of AIDS." Unpublished manuscript.

Krueger, L., Wood, R., Diehr, P., Maxwell, C. 1990. "Poverty and HIV Seropositivity: The Poor Are More Likely to Be Infected". AIDS 4(8): 811-14.

Lacey, C., Merrick, D., Bensley, D., Fairely, 1. Analysis of the Sociodemography of gonorrrhea in Leeds." *British Medical Journal* 314(l): 715-18.

Lewis, J., Arndt, C. 2000. The Macro Implications of HIV/AIDS in South Africa: a preliminary assessment. Paper presented at the International AIDS Economics Network Symposium. July 2000. Special submission to the *South African Journal of Economics.*

McCoy, C. B., Metsch, L., Inciardi, J., Anwyl, R., Wingerd, J., Bletzer, K. 1996. "Sex, Drugs and the Spread of HIV/AIDS in Belle Glade, Florida". *Medical Anthropology Quarterly* 10 (1): 83-93.

Merson, M., Dayton, J., O'Reilly, K. 2000. "Effectiveness of HIV Prevention Interventions in Developing Countries." AIDS. 14 (suppl. 2): S68-84.

Parker, R. G. 1998. 'Historic Overview of Brazil's AIDS Programmes and Review of the World Bank AIDS Project'. Family Health International/AIDSCAP. Processed. In Ainsworth, M., Semali, 1. "Who is most likely to die of AIDS? Socioeconomic correlates of adult deaths in Kagera Region, Tanzania." Cited in Ainsworth, M., Fransen, L, Over, M. (Eds). 1998, Confronting AIDS.- Evidence from the developing world. Selected background papers for the World Bank Policy Research Report, Confronting AIDS.- Public Priorities in a global epidemic. European Commission, Brussels, pp. 95-109.

Piot, P., Aggleton, P. 1998. "The Global Epidemic." AIDS Care, 10 (Suppl. 12) S200208.

Ram, S. 2000. A Summary of Resource Transfer Mechanisms. A discussion paper presented at the UNAIDS Workshop on the Role of Debt Relief in Financing National HIV/AIDS Programmes. Lilongwe, Malawi. November, 2000. Unpublished manuscript, pp. 24-26.

UNAIDS. 1999. Summary Booklet of Best Practice Collection. Issue 1. Geneva.

UNAIDS. 2000a. Report on the Global HIV/AIDS epidemic. Geneva, pp. 26-36.

UNAIDS. 2000b. Innovative Approaches to HIV Prevention. Selected Case Studies. Geneva. p. 6.

UNAIDS. 2000c. National AIDS Programmes.- A Guide to Monitoring and Evaluation. Geneva, pp. 26-27.

World Bank. 2000a. Poverty Reduction Sourcebook. http://www.worldbank.org/poverty. Accessed on 24 January 2001.

World Bank. 2000b. Project Appraisal Document for Proposed Credits in the amount of US$59.7 million and US$50 million, respectively, to the Federal Democratic Republic of Ethiopia and the Republic of Kenya in support of the first phase of the US$500 million multi-country HIV/AIDS Programme for the Africa Region. Washington, DC, pp. 65-79.

World Bank, 2000c. Costs of Scaling HIV Programme Activities to a National Level in Sub-Saharan Africa: Methods and Estimates. AIDS Campaign Team for Africa, pp. 1-5.

1. Burkina Faso, Uganda and United Republic of Tanzania.
2. In Africa: Benin, Cameroon, Central African Republic, Chad, Gambia, Ghana, Guinea, Guinea-Bissau, Kenya, Madagascar, Malawi, Mali, Mozambique, Niger Rwanda, Sao Tome and Principe, Senegal, United Republic of Tanzania, and Zambia. In Europe and Central Asia: Albania, FYR Macedonia, Georgia, Moldova, Tajikistan. In Latin America/Caribbean: Bolivia, Guyana, Honduras and Nicaragua. In Asia and the Pacific: Cambodia.
3. Source: World Bank website on HIPC: http://www.worldbank.org/hipc/about/hipcbr/hipcbr.htm.
4. In Africa: Benin, Burkina Faso, Cameroon, Gambia, Guinea, Guinea-Bissau, Madagascar Malawi, Mali, Mauritania, Mozambique, Niger Rwanda, Sao Tome and Principe, Senegal, Uganda, United Republic of Tanzania, Zambia. (Source: World Bank website, News release number 200111901S. December 22, 2000). In Latin American and Caribbean: Bolivia, Guyana, Honduras, Nicaragua. (Source: World Bank website, "The HIPC Initiative: Background and Progress Through December 2000 http://www.worldbank.org/hipc/progress-to-date/May99v3/may99v3.htm).

Fourteen

Getting Business Support for HIV/AIDS Control Programmes

Why AIDS should be a Business Concern

> "The threat of AIDS and the problems arising from it cannot be left to government and nongovernmental organisations alone. We are committed to the dire need to control the spread of AIDS and of discrimination against people with HIV-infection. The way forward is to accept that AIDS is a national problem at every employer's doorstep - it is a management problem."
>
> *A.L. Keembe, former Personnel Director, Barclays Bank of Zambia*

Since long AIDS prevention and care has been pitched to business on health terms by health experts, on the basis that 'dealing with AIDS in the workplace is good for workers'. Initially considered as a health problem, the health sector was at the forefront of epidemic control efforts. Experience has shown that both management and workers have a stake in the battle against AIDS and that all sectors need to participate right at the outset. Unquestionably, in the overall workplace context, management's response is a key factor in shaping the level and quality of company interventions. To mobilize the corporate sector's participation in a major way, management must participate as a stakeholder from the planning stage to implementation. Thailand has been relatively successful in getting cooperation from business, even though this initiative came at a late stage in the development of the epidemic. Thailand's success is due to continuing and determined efforts by the National AIDS Programme and nongovernmental organisations to create opportunities for key business leaders to contribute in a strategic and substantial fashion. Those in the business sector need to be impressed upon that their participation is essential in making a difference, not only to the larger national effort but also to their businesses.

1. AIDS is a low priority issue for business

Is AIDS a threat to business? The epidemic effects productivity, costs and markets and is thus clearly a bottom line issue. Lessons have been taken from many companies who have made HIV/AIDS their business. Over a decade of experience with AIDS at the workplace have brought out some compelling reasons why AIDS should be a business concern.

2. AIDS is already costing businesses, and these costs will continue without timely company interventions

In Kenya, an analysis showed that HIV/AIDS is costing companies an coverage of US$25 per employee every year, and costs would rise to an average of US$56 by 2005 if the rate of HIV infection were to go unchecked, whereas a comprehensive prevention programme would cost US$15 per employee.

A survey of a small company in Thailand found that AIDS was costing a loss of US$80,000 annually, on the other hand a prevention programme would cost US$11,500. A study in Bostwana by the Botswana Business Coalition on AIDS estimated that AIDS-related costs will soar from under 1 per cent of the wage bill to 5 per cent in six years time, due to the rapid rise in infection in the past few years.

AIDS results increase in health, pension, and welfare costs. Pension funds are being depleted by premature death, since payments into the funds are withdrawn early just as payments out increase. Insurance premiums rise as well. In Zimbabwe, for example, premiums on death-in service benefits quadrupled between 1992 and 1994 because of deaths due to AIDS. Some companies in Africa indicate a doubling in their health bills. In Zambia, one big company reported in 1995 that AIDS-related illness and deaths had cost them more than their total profits for the year.[1] Insufficient attention has been given to the cost impact of decreased productivity, obstruction in production due to absenteeism and increased demands for health care, which, taken all together, can take a serious toll on the profitability of a small business concern. Comprehensive workplace programmes and adequate HIV/AIDS policies can be implemented for a fraction of the amounts that would otherwise be spent because of AIDS-related illness and death. Managers want proof and estimates of the costs of AIDS and of prevention.

There are now tools available to measure the financial impact of the epidemic on company operations as well as the expenses of setting up and maintaining suitable HIV/AIDS programmes. The type and extent of on HIV/AIDS programme can be made to suit the needs and resources of each business.

3. Companies that participate - lending their name and resources—in fighting AIDS at the workplace and in their communities are rewarded with a positive public image.

The success of many businesses is largely dependent, on the goodwill of their customers and the communities from which they draw their workforces. Off late, the business sector has been supporting various social, civic, and health causes. These activities have been publicly accepted as an exercise of corporate citizenship and social responsibility. Multinational companies, like Levi Strauss, United Distillers, and Northwest Airlines who have ongoing AIDS education programmes are experiencing improved community relations and increased sales after being connected with AIDS support. United Distillers launched an AIDS awareness programme to market its Tanqueray gin. The company also established an ongoing series of Tanqueray-sponsored AIDS bicycle rides in the United States of America. This effort is now the biggest single AIDS fundraising event in the country. It has won the company an award for best cause-related marketing and made noticeable in the media and the community at large.

4. Employees are precious company asset and should be protected.

A Kenyan company manager said: "If you lose someone you've trained for twenty years, that's a great loss. Condoms and AIDS education cost peanuts."

Whether they are "white-" or "blue"-collar workers, a company's most valuable asset is its workforce. The capacity of employees to perform their jobs is a major management concern. Systems that provide for employee health and overall well being lead to higher productivity. Consistent productivity levels bring about national economic growth, which in turn affect general business climates.

The effect on the bottom line is heavily felt when technical staff fall ill. In Thailand, a large manufacturing conglomerate revealed that, inspite of abundant labour supply to replace employees, it would take 5-7 years for new employees in technical areas to equal the competence levels of their predecessors.

5. As the HIV/AIDS epidemic spreads, companies will face increasing employee-related issues.

Companies with rising numbers of employees who are HIV-positive are increasingly being involved in dealing with a variety of issues. Businesses need recruitment and employment policies that are fair and based on sound medical facts. These policies must be clearly spelled out and consistently applied. Employers need to know of the latest medical and scientific developments and to improve their policies according to new knowledge. Key policy areas include health care, work duties and performance, employee benefits (pensions, disability), recruitment, training, and costs.

As the AIDS threat continues to affect the workforce employers will increasingly need policies and mechanisms for dealing with personnel issues like absenteeism, sick leave, ill health, and early retirement. Furthermore, with more countries joining the expanded national AIDS programmes that will cover workplace issues, as have Uganda and the Philippines, the business sector will require to consider national and local regulations to protect the welfare of the workforce. It has become clear that procactive and transparent management action will be necessary in ensuring a fair and economically viable package of employee benefits, in the face of HIV/AIDS.

6. Businesses are now more globally linked politically, economically, and technologically.

Businesses can no longer overlook or deny the rising interdependence. The dynamics of economic globalization have brought about changes at the company level. Many local companies have become part of larger multinational groups or are connected to other businesses as suppliers, contractors or subsidiaries.

Increased mobility of workers within countries and across borders implies that migrant labour is an important feature of employment patterns, especially in agricultural, manufacturing and transportation industries. Advanced communication technologies and global media linkages increase information exchanges that influence attitudes and behaviours. These developments can change the nature or culture of a company's workforce, the customers for their products and services, and the communities in which they are active.[2] These socioeconomic changes have resulted in direct links with the risk and spread of HIV/AIDS. They may create or heighten circumstances that make a company's workforce vulnerable to HIV/AIDS or they may support the spread of information and attitudes that help in AIDS prevention.

Corporate Responses in Fight against AIDS

> "There is a clear role for business to play in these partnerships. Much more than just providing financial support, the business community, with its marketing and organisational skills, can bring a commercial efficiency to the delivery of health promotion messages to targeted audiences, whether they be young people in industrialized countries, or urban workers in emerging markets."
>
> *Sir Richard Sykes, CEO-Glaxo Welcome plc*

There are various examples of corporate responses with proven effectiveness in the fight against AIDS.

(i) Investing in AIDS programmes for companies and their stakeholders

Many companies have started funding in HIV/AIDS programmes for their employees; others have implemented education programmes for their employees' families, suppliers, and other members of the community. Workplace programmes often comprise training some staff members as "peer educators" to talk to colleagues about the risks of HIV and to discuss prevention methods, such as condom use and safer sex. Some companies supply condoms directly to their workers, or work with public or private distributors to ascertain condom availability and affordability in the market. Since HIV is spread faster by and to people suffering from untreated sexually transmitted diseases (STDs), some companies have trained educators to discuss about the signs and symptoms of these diseases.

Other companies make sure that STD treatment is available, either at their staff health services or from other health facilities. At the least , these efforts will aid risk-reducing behaviours among employees. This will help maintain a reliable supply of workers and encourage an economically vibrant community that will buy the company's goods and services.

(ii) Create association between business and local communities

Many companies may not be able to establish or carry out their own AIDS programmes owing to paucity of organisational, financial, and human resources. A company's size should not, however be a hindrance to progress. Collaborating with public health facilities to provide services for employees is a good option. In many countries, NGOs have well-established education, condom distribution and counselling programmes. Association between business and these organisations will be mutually beneficial financially. Larger, more financially secure companies have set up on "social investment" programmes where AIDS-related efforts in the external community have got benefits such as improvements in corporate image and healthier workforces.

An exemplary example of partnership is found in Thailand, where CARE (an NGO), the American International Assurances/ Thailand company, and the Ministry of Public Health have joined together to conduct AIDS Programmes going to thousands of factory workers and their surrounding communities.

The programmes use an array of materials and strategies like video-tapes, exhibitions, group workshops, comic books, and peer educators. The rapid assessment techniques and health communication skills of CARE, alongwith the financial and human resources of the other partners, has resulted in a lively, effective and ongoing AIDS initiative in the workplace.

(iii) Philanthropic initiatives

An increasing number of companies have extended their programmes into the wider society. Gifts or grants in the form of cash, equipment, technical assistance, or other resources have become part of corporate efforts for fighting the disease or benefiting specific affected groups. Some companies have, for instance, donated millions of dollars worth of equipment and technical support to assist AIDS organisations at local, national and international levels. Local companies have also indulged philanthropic giving, a typical response being in-kind assistance, such as free use of their facilities or equipment. Such donations are negligible cost to the company, but are often crucial to local AIDS efforts, and provide much-needed practical and moral support.

United Distillers offered major financial aid to the Confederation of Indian Industry's AIDS in the Workplace programme to help it reach its 3,500 industry members. Philanthropic contributions can give minimal financial advantage to a company but gives considerable social benefits by strengthening the company's standing in the community.

(iv) Promote cause-related marketing

Promoting AIDS messages while marketing product has become a popular strategy, specially among companies that have a wide consumer base. The Pilot Pen Corporation and Clairol Company include AIDS-related messages and the famous AIDS ribbon on their products. Other companies donate portions of their sales proceeds to support AIDS activities of national programmes and NGOs. These methods have yielded mutual benefits for companies and AIDS programmes — the wide retail base for the products carrying the AIDS messages has promoted greater public awareness of HIV/AIDS issues, while, from the companies' standpoint a positive image has been attained by associating their brands with a popular cause.

(v) Sustain the fight

Inspite of the continuing and growing threat of AIDS, some companies are decreasing their AIDS prevention efforts. A study of companies in the United States of America found that the number of corporations offering AIDS education has reduced 10 per cent in the past five years. The feeling that "AIDS is over" is simply incorrect. 16,000 people continue to be infected every day all over the world. There is no cure. Even though new drugs are being discovered that help lengthen lives, people in developing countries often have little or no access to these drugs. With 95 per cent of HIV infections now being reported in the developing world where 80 per cent of the productive sector live, there is a long battle to be won.

Because HIV/AIDS will seriously effect the economic growth, the business sector is a major stakeholder. Options chosen about how to act, indeed whether to act, to respond to the impact of HIV/AIDS, will make a difference to the immediate and long-term growth of individual businesses and the sector in general. HIV/AIDS programmes that have been effective have played a significant role for private sector participation. HIV/AIDS initiatives expand and are very effective when undertaken in partnership with the public sector. A national policy framework that gives opportunities and rewards for active, meaningful involvement of business in the national effort is a major constituent for this partnership.

An environment where incentives for action are extended and where the contributions of the business sector are acknowledged will drive HIV/AIDS higher on the business agenda. Corporations have an extremely rich array of resources in terms of skills, materials, and networks. Their participation in partnerships with government and nongovernment efforts will create a combination of resources whose impact will be felt far beyond national and corporate boundaries.

According to Nelson Mandela, President of the Republic of South Africa "All sectors and all spheres of society have to be involved as equal partners. We have to join hands to develop programmes and share information and research that will halt the spread of this disease and help develop support networks for those who are affected."

Thus, for effective action against AIDS, we need a strong partnership between the public and the private sector. Businesses should give their expertise and provide financial aid to the national AIDS programme. In return, the national AIDS programme should help create a social climate that is conducive to private-sector action, an environment that enables businesses to participate in AIDS prevention and care.

References

1. From the UNAIDS, Family Health International, and the Organisation of African Trade Union Unity (OATUU) Joint Consultation Workshop on Workplace Actions in East and Southern Africa, July 20-22, 1998.
2. From Prince of Wales Business Leaders Forum, p. 8.

Fifteen

Health Rights of Migrants'

The world is moving at a very fast pace. The twentieth century saw a tremendous pace of development in all the sectors of the economy. The development was largely possible due to interchange of skills and technologies which has been a catalyst for change. This interchange has been largely due to education, employment, conferences and forums, trade agreements, etc. In pursuance of the above there were large numbers of population that migrated within the country and an equally large number going outside World Bank. Figures reveal that the country in 1995 at least 125 million people resided outside their country of origin.[1] Every year, over one million people emigrate permanently and nearly as many seek asylum. However, if we include short-term visitors in the definition of mobile people, then there are over one billion international travellers every year. In some tourist destination countries, the annual number of short-term visitors even exceeds the resident population.[2] While including in-country mobility; figures would probably reach the two billion people mark.

This study addresses some of the issues involved in relation to the rights of migrants to health. These issues revolve around two main themes: (a) Definition of migrant, and (b) what is included in the relation to right to health. Haour-Knipe and Rector[3] devoted several pages to their definition(s). As summarized by Decosas and Adrien:[4] "Migrants may be defined by their legal status or ethnicity, or migration can be categorized using parameters of duration, motivation, and distance. If we exclude short-term visitors (tourists, for example), the most important categories are labour migration, refugee migration, resettlement migration, internal migration, and commuting."

Lurie[5] uses a different approach: "most studies simply classify people as either 'migrants' or 'non-migrants'. In reality the situation is considerably more compels; there are in fact many different types of migration, and each type may carry with it different risk factors. In addition, people's migration status is likely to change several times over the course of their lives."

Each country uses its own definitions in its rules of how to categories of travellers and migrants. International law differentiates between people who are and are not national, e.g., citizens, foreignness, immigrants, and recognizes other special categories, e.g. refugees, asylum-seekers, migrant workers. Here we will utilize a definition of migrants that encompasses all aspects of mobility in any population. We will focus on people who are presently crossing or have crossed borders at some time. These include people mobile for professional and educational reasons, as well as youth. We do not include refugees (covered elsewhere) and ethnic minority communities (for whom the issues may be quite different) in this study.

The issues for refugees are similar to those for all migrants, but the basic problems are usually exaggerated. As noted by many authors, including Forrest:[6] "forced or unplanned migration due to civil or natural disaster presents significant stress on population health status and nutrition, medical care and public health systems, favouring emergence and dissemination of disease." Also included in this study are key existing laws, policies and best practices with respect to the right of migrants to health, and associated care, treatment, support and prevention, particularly with respect to HIV/AIDS/STD and reproductive health matters. While poising this study the framework of existing laws and policies are referred to while addressing ethical and economic dimensions, and while considering the effects of globalization and the consequences of policies for migrant health.

World Figures of Migrant Population

According to the recent International Labor Organisation (ILO) Reports[7] over 90 million people (migrant workers and their families) are currently residing, legally or illegally, in a country other than there by own. This lower estimate, compared with the 1995 estimate by the World Bank of 125 million people living outside their countries of origin, excludes people who had officially changed their original nationality.[8] Table 1 below (taken from the ILO report) breaks down this figure by region.

TABLE - 1
ESTIMATE OF THE NUMBER OF NON-NATIONALS BY MAJOR REGION IN 1995, EXCLUDING ASYLUM-SEEKERS AND REFUGEES
(in millions)[9]

Region	*Economically active*	*Dependants*	*Total*
Africa	6-7	12-14	18-21
North America	8	8-10	16-18
Central and South America	3-5	4-7	7-12
South, South-East & East Asia	2-3	3-4	5-7
West Asia (Arab States)	6	2-3	8-9
Europe	11-13	15-17	26-30
Overall Totals	36-42	44-55	80-97

Countries function at the same time as senders and receivers of migrants. Whereas some countries may be major senders of migrants, some countries are major receivers, and in many cases, countries may be both sizeably senders and receivers of migrants. According to the ILO in 1990, over 100 countries were major senders or receivers of migrant labor, with 68 countries listed as major receivers, 56 as major senders, and 24 as both a sending and receiving country.[10] Countries noted to be among the new major receiving countries were Italy, Japan, Malaysia, venezuela, Bangladesh, Egypt and Indonesia contributed in terms of being the new major senders.

Striking Revealations between Migrant Patterns

While addressing the problem of assessing number of migrants, certain striking revealation have been made.

(a) About 7 million (3 per cent) of the United States population were born in Mexico. These included 2.7 million unauthorized migrants. Between 80 and 90 per cent of these migrants are male, mostly single or unaccompanied, between 15 and 34 year of age. (1996)

(b) In a region of Ziguinichor, Senegal, 82 per cent of men aged between 20 and 40 migrate each year. Movement within and between countries may be disproportionately heavy in some regions.

(c) Contrary to the perception that a typical migrant is male, the ILO Migrant Workers Report notes that about half the entire 1999 migrant population worldwide is female[11] While drawing the attention of government to the particular vulnerability to exploitation and abuse of women migrant workers:

(d) Migration and gender issues are inextricably connected. As Singhanetra-Renard[12] notes "Since women migrants almost invariably possess lesser bargaining power and legal rights than locals and particularly local men, the role of migration in the victimization of women, and thus, the spread of HIV infection, cannot be ignored." In addition to this, a particular risk for women migrants is the large scale and syndicated trafficking of women worldwide. These women, who include very young and from economically depressed countries or communities, may be forced into sex work, very often including unprotected sex.[13]

"No longer only to be found among accompanying family members, women now make up an increasing proportion of migrant workers: for instance, nearly half a million Sri Lankan women are working in the Middle East, while there are 12 women for every man among migrants form the Philippines to other Asian countries... The Committee notes in particular the increasing tendency to 'import' women migrant workers for commercial — including sexual — exploitation through arranged marriages with foreigners or by getting them to sign contracts of employment that look tempting but rarely reflect the real situation. Their vulnerability lies principally in the fact that they are employed abroad and hence outside the legal protection of their country of origin, but is also due to the fact that they often hold jobs for which there is little protection under social legislation: domestic workers, manual workers (in agriculture, factories or export processing zines), hostesses or entertainers in night clubs of cabarets, etc. Their situation is made worse by the lack of autonomy and the strong relationship of subordination that are typical of the jobs usually held by these workers; added to this is the fact that these women are usually young and poor, living in fear of losing their jobs, having had to leave their families in their countries of origin, do not speak the language of the country of employment, are unaware that they have rights that are being infringed, and usually do not know where to go for help."

Approaches to Social Policies Involving-Migrants

Specific pressures are often placed on workers who migrate. A WHO Background Paper on Long Term Travel Restrictions and HIV/AIDS[14] notes: Countries generally adopt three approaches to social policies involving migrants as noted by ILO:

"Newly industrialised States may welcome migrant workers. But at the same time, they may seek to prevent such workers from acquiring long-term settlement rights, so they can be sent home if they cease to be economically useful because of changing labour demands or because of age, illness or disability. Fixed term employment contracts and work permits may be imposed on migrant workers to ensure that they provide the employer and host country with a 'rotating stock of temporary labour'.[15]

(i) countries who accept migrants for permanent settlement on entry, like Australia and Canada, are more likely to favour social policies aiming at both social integration and multiculturalism'.

(ii) countries issuing permanent resident status after several years in the country are more possible to focus on 'assimilations' policies.

(iii) countries viewing migrant's primarily as temporary workers are expected to favour voluntary repatriation and reintegration assistance. For example, Germany does not admit migrants for permanent settlement on entry. It devotes its social policy objectives towards encouraging voluntary repatriation through the institution of the Coordinating Agency for Promoting the Reintegration of Foreign Workers. Germany ranks among one of the main migratory destinations in Europe. Almost 10 per cent of the population comprises of migrants. However, if those living and working irregularly were included, the percentage would be significantly higher.

There are also three types of provision relating to illegal immigration in national laws and regulations:

(a) those directed at migrant workers in an irregular situation:
(b) those aimed at punishing persons who organize or facilitate clandestine or illicit migrations; and
(c) those penalizing the illegal recruitment and employment of migrant workers.

The ILO[16] noted with concern that steps taken fight against clandestine movements of migrants were supposed to be targeted at the demand for clandestine labor rather than the supply; but, in a reality, sanctions against migrant in an irregular situation are very common, both in sending and receiving countries. Sometimes these sanctions may be aimed at the dependants of illegal migrants rather than the migrants themselves: for example, an Amendment in California, United States, in 1996, which attempts to discourage irregular immigration by preventing children of undocumented migrants from state-funded education (from kindergarten to university).

The CIS (Commonwealth of Independent States) had more than 900,000 refugees, 1.1 million internally displaced persons, and 4.2 million repatriates during 1989-1996. Due to environmental degradation there were hundreds of thousands of ecological migrants. To add to this legal and illegal transit migration increased. Approximately about 500,000 to one million illegal migrants, particularly Afghans, Iranians, and Iraqi Kurds, are living in the Russian Federation alone. Emigration, largely to the CIS, has increased dramatically from countries with continuous armed conflicts, such as Armenia, Georgia, and Tajikistan. With few exceptions, the largest number of current migrants have shifted residence for economic reasons, and in contrast with most other such movements, the age composition of the migrant population is very similar to that of the general population.

Causes of Population Movement

According to the UNAIDS Technical Update on Migration and HIV/AIDS[17], population movement has increased in recent years because of:

(a) greater availability of inexpensive air transport;

(b) opening up of once-closed borders, specially in Eastern European countries and the Commonwealth of Independent States (CIS), South Africa, and Economic Free zones along China's east coast;

(c) rising international trade and commerce, as well as deregulation of trade practices and promotion of regional free trade; and

(d) increasing awareness of these imbalances even by the populations in poorer countries.

A considerable amount of global movement of peoples is expected to increase during the coming years. Migration has always been mainly due to the desire for greater prosperity and/or escape from civil or natural disasters. By the year 2000, only some 20 per cent of the world's population will live in developed countries, and economic polarization may result in increased migration. Similarly, as noted by Gellert[18] environmental problems associated with increasing industrialization such as rising sea levels from global warming, desertification and deforestation may result in substantial increases in the numbers of ecological refugees. With the growth in the numbers of countries following policies to lower immigration,[19] combined with this external pressure of increased global movement, the numbers and proportion of illegal and marginalized migrants in many countries can also be expected to increase considerably in times to come.

Ethnic Distances and Access to Health

Health has been well acknowledged as a fundamental human right. The Constitution of the World Health Organisation defines health as "a state of complete physical, mental and social well-being and not merely the absence of disease or infirmity." In respect of non-citizens, most countries have determined their obligations in terms of essential care or care in emergency situations, with this policy being interpreted in different ways in different countries. Even with respect to officially accepted migrant workers, special arrangements to ensure real equity in access to health (compared with nationals are not very often put in place. In this perspective there have been a number of documenting the reduced access to health care and the health consequences for migrants in many parts of the world.[20]

Bollini and Siem contend that the poor health outcomes observed are connected the lower entitlements for migrants and ethnic groups in the receiving countries.[21] They note:

> "Not only are they exposed to poor working and living conditions, which are *per se* determinants of poor health, but they also have reduced access to health care for a number of political, administrative and cultural reasons which are not necessarily present for the native population, and which vary in different societies and for different groups. Language, different concepts of health and disease, or the presence of racism are examples of such selective barriers."[22]

Though the 'migrants' do not form a uniform group. Bollini and Siem opine that the general trend to poor health outcomes may differ from one group of migrants to another and for individuals within a group - however, the general statement is valid in most parts of the world. It has been noted that, the tendency for migrants to have less access to health care and resultant poorer health status is more in case of recent arrivals or for 'groups' who are otherwise more socially backward in the host country (e.g. North Africans in France, Bangladesh is in the United kingdom, Indonesians in Malaysia).

Tan[23] offers the term 'ethnic distance' to explain the elements of cultural differences and risk inherent in moves from one country to another even where the same sending and host countries are involved. In a case study of two nationals of the Philippines moving to Hong Kong for work purposes, Tan notes that the ethnic distance for the young Filipina from a small village going to work as a domestic helper in Hong Kong is much greater than that for a young Filipino male executive also going to Hong Kong to take up a job with a multinational corporation. In cases where the sending and host countries are highly different in cultural values, this ethnic distance can be even more increased.

Migrant workers having health problems often return to their home countries due to financial needs, lack of proper immigration documents and ill health – this return is increasingly, being related to HIV/AIDS. Many countries have now witnessed large numbers of nationals returning to die among their relatives or original communities. This brings to notice the delicate balance required by governments and policy-makers between acknowledging that migrants may be more vulnerable to infection in their new environment, while avoiding, tendency to migrants for bringing HIV with them into the country/ community. A recent initiative by - Greece's Ministry of Health and Welfare appears to be a good example of how to achieve this balance. Greece is promoting an information programme with the slogan: "Taking Care of Migrants' Health at the Same Time as Our Own".

The above instance demonstrates only rare instances of such approaches. According to CARAM-Asia there have been a number of violations of human rights of migrant workers that have an effect on their health and well-being. It has been found that many migrant workers in South and South-east Asia experience miserable working conditions, such as working 12 hours or more a day for six or seven days a week; insufficient food and un-healthy sleeping quarters provided by the employers, and other breaches. They note that sexual and physical abuses are yet other occupational risks many migrant workers have to face. All these severe and abusive conditions of life and work can directly have an impact on the immune system, and thus result in migrants becoming immuno-compromised to various types of diseases and infections including HIV.

National statistics on disability and mortality rates underestimate the outcomes of semi-skilled and unskilled migrant workers - for example Egger[24] et al. found that Swiss data left out on significant numbers of these groups who had suffered occupational accidents and related disabilities but had then left Switzerland when they were too disabled or sick to work. Even though the migrant workers are chosen for their good health and ability to work (the 'healthy migrant effect'), there is proof that later in life many end up with a substantial amount of disability (the 'exhausted migrant effect'). However, specific actions can be surprisingly effective: for example, Bollini and Siem[25] note that pregnancy outcomes (stillbirth and peri-natal mortality) in Sweden were slightly better for foreign women that for Swedish women, in spite of the fact that many come from countries (notably Turkey) where peri-natal mortality rates were very high compared with Sweden. They understand that this may be due to the fact that, as reported by Sachs[26], considerable attention has been given in Sweden to leaving about cultural differences in mother and child care between Swedish and Turkish women, and to the provision of culturally suited services.

Cairo Conference: Conclusions and Recommendations

An area of common neglect in respect of migrants' health needs is that of reproductive rights. The 1994 Cairo Conference redefined sexual and reproductive health with in moral principles. The Conference acknowledged that:

(a) there had been failure to address people's reproductive health requirements. This was a matter of human rights and social justice.

(b) people had the freedom to make free and informed decisions about their reproductive lives;

(c) people have a right to information and care that will help them to protect their ours as well as their families health, and

(d) people have a right to benefit from scientific advance in health care.

Dr. Gro Harlem Brundtland, Director-General of WHO, has stated that "defining reproductive ill-health as not only a health issue but as a matter of social justice provides a legal and political basis for governments to act."[27] She noted that

> "between 5 and 15 per cent of the global burden of disease is associated with failures to address reproductive health needs. This burden hits people - particularly women - in the prime of their life, it hits when their potential, responsibilities, and productivity are at their highest. Globally, among women of reproductive age, more than 20 per cent of total years of healthy life lost are due to three main groups of reproductive health conditions -

> sexually transmitted diseases including HIV/AIDS, material mortality and morbidity and reproductive tract cancers. A further 10 per cent healthy years of life are lost due to conditions affecting the newborn."

Stray incidents show that migrant women are affected disproportionately. Anther major drawback in most countries is attention to the issue of migration and psychosocial health. As stated by Carballo and Siem,

> "The culture shock that often accompanies initial contact with a new sociocultural system can be psychologically complex and involve far more than the simple negation of access to local health and social services. Social integration and then acculturation is a complicated process involving linguistic, social, cultural and conceptual transference processes that can denude migrants of everything they have previously been used to and which may have provided the basis for their identity. The migration of people from rural and often very traditional communities.....to major industrial cities can equally involve a confirmation of widely different values, expectations, and ways of life. It is a process pregnant with psychological and psychosomatic problems which have remained poorly understood and even less well addressed by receiving countries."[28]

Other than the specific issues, and as has been noted in many countries, the ongoing attitude towards immigration and 'foreigners' (or subgroups of 'foreigners') influence the response of the health care system to their special needs.

Routes to Mobility and Risk Perception

Several studies have shown an association between human mobility and increased risk of HIV infection. For example, Chardin reported that while migrants constitute 6 per cent of the population of France, 14 per cent of the reported cases of AIDS occur among migrants.[29] However, as Decosas and Adrien[30] note, there are difficulties faced by many epidemiological surveys as they often lead to a focus on migrants rather than on the factors increasing risk in mobile populations. It has be deduced that being a migrant, in and of itself, is not a risk factor; it is the activities undertaken during the migration process that are the actual risk factors.

People move for all kinds of reasons, these include – business, pleasure, escaping political persecution or armed conflicts, in search of a better life for themselves and their children. This movement need not involve the crossing of any borders: in China, for example, about 100 million people are considered mobile between rural and urban areas, and from one urban area to another. More so India also has a large number of rural to urban migrants in search of livelihood, education or for a better life.

There have been an increased number of individuals in a number of countries have become bi-local or even multi-local, within a country or in a different country than the country of origin. Specially for students but increasingly for many others, a pattern of circular mobility is part of life. As Singhanetra- Renard observes in regard to Thailand, "daily commuting, seasonal migration, periodic, short- and long-term circulation are undertaken by both the rural and urban population for employment, education, entertainment, as well as for other socio-cultural reasons."[31]

People's mobility tends to follow opportunities, taking place more commonly form rural to urban areas and/or from poorer to richer countries. But it surely can be a two-way traffic: migrants who do well in the city or in another country will often go back to their places of origin bringing evidence of the good life. And, while moving may increase risk and lead to people engaging in higher vulnerable behavior, it is by no means axiomatic. For example, as Tan[32] writes:

> "rural women may not be able to break out of their low social status if they stay in their village. Their future is limited to an early marriage, often with little bargaining power and little support for reproductive and sexual health. Migrating to cities is still an option for social mobility and could actually mean a better quality of life and health. A shift to an urban environment, where sexuality-related issues can be more openly discussed, may also be beneficial."

One of the features of mobile individuals, particularly those who are voluntarily mobile, is that they are risk-takers—they are risking the fact that a different environment will be advantageous to them. This concept of risk-taking may then lead on to choice they make in their private lives. At times people are able to move with their entire families. However, for most labour migration, this is not the case. In Asia, there is a large regional movement of female workers who provide services of domestic help; in many other parts of the world, there is single sex migration predominantly male to work in industries such as mining, construction and agriculture.

The changed environment may lead to increased personal vulnerability: perhaps separated form family, from a regular sex partner, in single-sex housing, and with the stresses and risks associated with the migration process. For some, there is a strong need for money to buy necessities or on which to subsist while waiting for employment. For others, the anonymity of being an alien, especially in transit areas, can increase sexual indulgence. Similarly, loneliness, frustration and peer pressure together with easier access to drugs can make it hard for some to resist injecting drugs. More so, there may be drug dealers exploiting this vulnerability. Sometimes, moving may be undertaken so that the individual may indulge in what might be illegal or considered shameful in their own neighborhood. For example, CARAM-Asia has noted that "thousands of poor Vietnamese women come to Cambodia to earn [money] by engaging in sex work...one third of the commercial sex workers reported being born in Vietnam.[33]

In many instances moving is related to a perceived upward social mobility. Singhanetra-Renard[34] documents that ways to social mobility for rural Thai can include:

- "Secure salaried employment in government, service, manufacturing or business enterprises even at the lower end of the hierarchy such as janitor, cleaner, or gardener, since it signifies a connection with city dwellers who have position, politically, financially or socially;
- Professional employment such as police, soldier, nurse, or secretarial job or any other position, including informal sector work, in which employees wear uniforms;
- Employment in enterprises which symbolize modernity

or Western influence such as golf courses, discos, coffee shops, cocktail lounges, and karaoke bars;

- Marriage to a government official, Chinese, or others who have position, wealth, or connections."35

Sighanetra-Renard, however, also notes that pathways to social mobility differ for men and for woman, and that women will "often take a short-cut through commercial sex-work."

The numbers and proportion of communities affected by migration are substantial for instance, surveys in Africa found that between one-fifth and one-third of men and women reported living apart from their regular sexual partner, with one of two major after effects-sexual abstinence or having multiple partners.[36]

This may lead to a consequence such as reported by Kane et al: a study of the nexus between migration and HIV status of Senegalese villagers found that 27 per cent of the men who had previously travelled in other African countries and 11.3 per cent of the wives of such men were HIV-infected. In contrast, from the control group (414 people) who had not moved outside Senegal in the previous ten years, only one man and one woman were HIV+.[37] In Mexico, 25 per cent people reported to be living with AIDS in rural regions have a history of temporary migration to the United States.

References

1. World Bank. Workers in an Integrating World: world development Report 1995. Oxford University Press, 1995.
2. Hendricks A. "The right to freedom of movement and the (un) lawfulness of AIDS/HIV specific travel restrictions from a European perspective." Nordic journal of International law 59: Fasc. 2/3, 1990.
3. Haour- Knipe M and Rector R. Crossing borders: migration, ethnicity and AIDS. London, Taylor & Francis, 1996.
4. Decosas J and Adrian A. "Migration and HIV". AIDS 1997, 11 (suppl. A): 577-584.
5. Lurie M, Garnett G, Abdool Karim S, Strum W, Wilkinson D, and Williams B. Research Protocol. Migration and the Spread of HIV and Other Sexually Transmitted Diseases in South Africa : Interlocking Urban and Rural Cohort Studies. January 1998.
6. Forrest DM. "Control of Imported Communicable Diseases: Preparation and Response". Canadian Journal of Public Health, Vol. 87, No. 6. November-December 1996, p. 369.

7. ILO. Migrant Workers, International Labour Conference, 87th Session 1999, Report III (Part 1B). Geneva, 1999.
8. The lower estimate by the ILO may be due to naturalized citizens being excluded as part of migrant populations, but included within the World Bank scope of people living outside their country of origin.
9. The estimate refers to foreign passport-holders, not to foreign-born persons because the latter include an unknown proportion of naturalized persons who no longer hold the nationality of their country of origin. The figures given here include both regular migrants and migrants whose status may be irregular as regards entry, stay or economic activity.
10. ILO. Migrant Workers, 1999, op. cit., p. 4.
11. *Ibid*, p. 105.
12. Singhanetra-Renard A. "Population movement and the AIDS epidemic in Thailand", Paper presented at the IUSSP Seminar on Sexual Subcultures and Migration in the Era of AIDS/STDs, Bangkok, Thailand, March 1994, p. 14.
13. Ybanez RFC. "Breaking Borders: Migration and HIV/AIDS" AIDS action, Issue 40, July-September 1998.
14. WHO. Background Paper: Long Term Travel Restriction and HIV/AIDS. WHO Global Programme on AIDS, October 1994, p. 4.
15. Papademetriou DG. "International migration in North America and Western Europe: trends and consequences" In Appleyard R (ed). International migration today: Volume 1, trends and prospects. Paris, UNESCO, 1998, as quoted in WHO Background paper, *ibid*.
16. ILO. Migrant Workers, 1999, Op. cit., p. 130.
17. UNAIDS. Technical Update on Migration and HIV/AIDS, UNAIDS, 2000.
18. Gellert GA. "International Migration and Control of Communicable Diseases", Soc. Sci. Med. Vol. 37 , No. 12, 1993, pp. 1489-1499.
19.
20. See, for example, European Project AIDS and Mobility: AIDS & STDs and Migrants, Ethnic Minorities and other Mobile Groups; the State of Affairs in Europe, de Putter J(ed.). June 1998; Haour-Knipe M and Rector R. Crossing borders: migration, ethnicity and AIDS. London, Taylor & Francis, 1996; ILO: Migrant Workers, International Lobour Conference, 87th Session 1999, Report III (Part 1B). Geneva, 1999; Mishra SI, Conner RF and Magana JR (eds.) AIDS. Crossing Borders: The Spread of HIV Among Migrant Latinos. Colorado, Westview Press, 1996.
21. Bollini P and Siem H. "No Real Progress towards Equity: Health of Migrants and Ethnic Minorities on the eve of the Year 2000", Soc. Sci. Med. Vol. 41, No. 6, pp 819-828, 1995.
22. *Ibid.*, p. 821.
23. Tan M. " Migration and Risk", AIDS action, Issue 40, July-September 1998, p. 2.
24. Egger M, Minder CE and Smith GD. "Health inequalities and migrant workers in Switzerland", Lancet 816, Sept 29, 1990.
25. Bollini and Seim, op. cit., p. 823.
26. Sachs L. Evil Eye or Bacteria. Turkish Migrants and Swedish Health Care, Stockholm Studies in Social Anthropology, University of Stockholm, 1993.

27. World Health Organisation. Statement by Dr Gro Harlem Brundtland, Director- General, World Health Organisation, ICPD + 5 Forum, The Hague, 8-12 February 1999, p. 6.
28. Crossing Borders, op. cit. p. 36.
29. Chardin C. "Access to new treatments for migrants living with HIV and AIDS: The Policy Maker's Point of View - the Political and Juridical Situation in France" in Access to New Treatments for Migrants Living with HIV and AIDS - Second Annual Seminar, National Focal Points, European Project AIDS & Mobility, Clarke K and Bröring G (eds) October 1999, p. 15.
30. Decosas and Adrien, 1997, op. cit., p. 578.
31. Singhanetra-Renard, op. cit., p. 2.
32. Tan M. op cit, p. 2.
33. Coordination of Action Research on AIDS and Migration, op. cit., p. 20.
34. Singhanetra-Renard, op. cit., p. 9.
35. *Ibid*, p. 9.
36. Cleland J and Ferry B. Sexual behaviour and AIDS in the developing world. London, Taylor & Francis, 1996, as cited in Haour- Knipe M and Aggleton P, "Social enquiry and HIV/AIDS", Critical Public Health, Vol. 8, No. 4, 1998, p. 261.
37. Kane F, Alary M, Ndoye I et al. "Temporary expatriation is related to HIV-1 infection in rural Senegal." AIDS 1993, 7:1261-1265.

Index

D

S

T

U

V